"Oh, great, it's Mr. Sunshine." She said this under her breath, but when she peeked out from behind a clump of leaves, she could tell Chris had heard her.

"You are aware that you're late for your appointment, yes?"

Susannah clenched her teeth. She was hanging like tinsel in the bush, but she knew she couldn't be more than a minute or two late.

"Technically, I am on the premises. And arrived perfectly on time."

"Yes, but the council tends to object when I castrate animals in the parking lot. Do you need help?"

He helped extricate her and Hendrix from the bush, half tangling himself up with her at one point when Hendrix realized he'd been thwarted.

She turned back to Chris. "Thank you."

"Training going well, then?"

He was thoroughly ticking her off now. She narrowed her eyes at him, giving him her best glare, and he mirrored

So annoying. He looks ̶

"Well, there's no point your time, then, is there up and down, as if to se̶ ̶̶ ̶̶ ̶̶ ̶̶ ̶̶ ̶̶ ̶̶ ̶̶ ̶̶ ̶ ̶ ̶ ̶ to his stupidly arrogant and rather hot body.

Dear Reader,

Thank you for reading! I hope you loved spending time in Puddle Lake with its zany inhabitants!

Big thanks go out to Harlequin. It's one big family and I'm super proud to be a part of it.

Special thanks for the Doberman advice goes to thriller queen Lisa Hall. Thank you for sharing your stories about your lovely dogs! I hope you like Hendrix as much as I do.

Writing about a hospice was very special. I think we can all agree that cancer has affected most of us at some point, and highlighting the work of these amazing, caring professionals was very important to me. My own local hospice, Wakefield Hospice, has cared for many over the years, and funding is very limited. Taking part in a six-mile charity walk in 2020, I saw firsthand how dedicated and vital hospice workers are. I am in awe of the professionals I write about. If you are one and are reading this, thanks for what you do.

Lastly, thanks go out, of course, to my friends and family. Love you more.

Thank you so much, dear readers, for coming with me on this journey. I can't wait for our next trip!

Rachel Dove

FALLING FOR THE VILLAGE VET

RACHEL DOVE

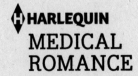

HARLEQUIN
MEDICAL
ROMANCE

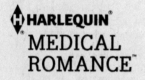

HARLEQUIN®
MEDICAL
ROMANCE™

Recycling programs
for this product may
not exist in your area.

ISBN-13: 978-1-335-73730-4

Falling for the Village Vet

Copyright © 2022 by Rachel Dove

For questions and comments about the quality of this book,
please contact us at CustomerService@Harlequin.com.

Harlequin Enterprises ULC
22 Adelaide St. West, 41st Floor
Toronto, Ontario M5H 4E3, Canada
www.Harlequin.com

Printed in U.S.A.

Rachel Dove is a tutor and romance/rom-com author from West Yorkshire in the UK. She lives with her husband and two sons, and dreams of a life where housework is done by fairies and she can have as many pets as she wants. When she is not writing or reading, she can be found walking her American cocker spaniel, Oliver, in the great outdoors or dreaming of her next research trip away with the family.

Books by Rachel Dove

Harlequin Medical Romance

Fighting for the Trauma Doc's Heart
The Paramedic's Secret Son

Visit the Author Profile page at Harlequin.com.

I dedicate this book to Carly Byrne, my amazing editor. Thank you for believing in my writing from day one and pushing me to be a better writer. You are an inspiration!

A special mention to Lisa Hall, thriller queen, for her Doberman insights.

Praise for
Rachel Dove

"I found Rachel Dove's interpretation broke that mold and I enjoyed the realistic way in which she painted the personalities. All in all, the well-crafted characters plus the engaging story had me emotionally invested from the start. Looking forward to reading more of Rachel's work."

—*Goodreads* on
Fighting for the Trauma Doc's Heart

CHAPTER ONE

'I JUST DIDN'T know what to do, Doctor—he's just not himself. He's so listless, and he doesn't eat like he used to.'

Mrs Chan looked mournfully at her beloved other half, who looked back at her glassy-eyed and defeated. This was the hardest part of the job. It took a lot of compassion, a lot of heart, and tact. These were all things, unfortunately, of which this particular doctor was in short supply at the moment. He found himself feeling nothing but irritation towards Mrs Chan; he brushed the feeling aside as best he could most days but he could still feel it there. Bubbling under the surface. He had thought that moving to a brand-new place would have lifted his mood a lot more than it had. He just felt angry and sad in a new place instead. Sure, Puddle Lake was a very pretty village, but he still felt the same as he did in the city. Angry, frustrated. He tried to smile at Mrs Chan, but it came out more like a toothless grimace.

'The problem, Mrs Chan, is that Gustav here is rather…well, he's rather fat, isn't he?' Mrs Chan's jaw dropped, but he had started talking now and he needed to get his point across. 'Now, I don't want you to misunderstand me, Mrs Chan. I know you love your cat. Unfortunately, he loves his food too, but a cat is incapable of saying no. He doesn't get onto the scales in the morning and worry about his waistline. If the food is there he will eat it. If he goes round to the neighbours and begs for food, he will eat that too. This is what cats do.'

Mrs Chan was looking decidedly miffed still, but her expression had softened.

'It's a common misconception that the giving of treats to pets is love. Sadly, often this is not the case. Dogs, cats, lots of animals need a balanced diet and it is the job of the owner to provide it. What I'm saying, Mrs Chan, is that he needs to stay on his diet food and nothing else. That's the way to show him love. He's an active cat but he's miserable because he can't move. He wants to lick himself and be able to reach all the parts that he could reach before and no longer can.' Gustav looked at the vet and meowed mournfully.

It's okay, buddy, Chris thought. *I've got your back. Just lay off the treats. Buy a little kitty treadmill.*

'So, what are you saying, Dr Jennings?'

'Basically, if you love little Gustav here any more with those treats of yours, then he's likely to run through his nine lives a lot quicker.'

Mrs Chan's incensed look told him that he'd gone too far, but in truth he would have gone further to stop the woman from feeding the poor feline to death. He did care about the patients he had, even if he was indifferent to everything else.

'I think we might need to speak to Dr Ingham, instead.' She looked him up and down, and her expression told him in no uncertain times that his curt words had fallen on deaf ears. 'Does Cheryl have his number?'

Chris resisted the urge to roll his eyes. The second week on the job, and all but one of his patients had asked the same question. He suddenly missed his old practice, the rapport he'd built up with the families of the animals he'd spent years caring for. It was a different world there, familiar and comfortable. He didn't have time for this, with his full clinic. He sighed inwardly, focusing back onto Mrs Chan's disapproving face.

'I am sure that Dr Ingham would agree with my diagnosis, given that he was the one to put Gustav on the diet food, but you are of course free to get a second opinion. I am afraid, however…' He wasn't at all, but he had to at least try to keep up the thin veneer of being polite. Somewhat misunderstood even. 'Dr Ingham is on vacation at the moment, and he's not taking calls. Cheryl is of course taking messages, for when he's back.' Dr Ezekiel Ingham, the man who had offered Chris the practice here, was probably three sheets to the wind on the cruise ship with his family right now and wouldn't give a fig about Mrs Chan or Gustav.

Maybe I should have done that, he thought to himself grumpily. *Sold up and just travelled, instead of…well, this.* 'I'll see you and Gustav out, Mrs Chan. You can settle your bill in Reception.'

Gustav was already sitting back in his little carrier, throwing Chris a scowl that matched his owner's. Mrs Chan huffed, picking up her rather portly cat and giving the vet her dirtiest final look, and left the room. Poor Cheryl. He could already hear Mrs Chan moaning about his bedside manner, and his new receptionist giving out the usual apologetic patter that she had taken to since he arrived. It was all he'd heard. He felt a little guilty, but he couldn't help his moods. He wasn't interested in being a polite functioning human. He was always there for his patients. Work was always something he excelled at. Now that it was his *only* focus, it had only honed his skills further. At the moment, he got dressed of a morning, fed himself, paid his bills and showed up to the new practice. That was enough for now, surely?

The front door to the surgery slamming shut gave him an inkling that perhaps it wasn't. Sighing heavily, he washed his hands in the sink and started to prepare for the next client. He was just reaching for the door handle to call the next patient when it was barged open by a rather dirty and eager-looking snout. The dog, looking as if he had bathed in mud, bounded into the room, his lead flying in the air as the mad Doberman dashed around the room. It took all of five seconds before the dog caught the scent of where he was, and he tried to bound right back out of the door. The lead thwacked Chris in the leg as he passed, and, in the waiting area, he could hear a woman's panicked shouting.

'Hendrix, you daft dog! Calm down!' The woman entered the room, blocking off the exit to the dog with a well-placed knee. Hen-

drix was overjoyed to see the woman, whoever she was, and Chris was still rubbing at
his trousered leg, where a nice red welt was
now showing on his ankle from the whipping
of the metal dog lead. 'Sorry, I'm so sorry,
he's a bit...well...bouncy.'

'Indeed.' Chris grabbed at the lead and the
big brown hound came to a stop at his feet.
'Hendrix, eh?'

'Yeah.' The woman, red-faced from wres-
tling with the dog, beamed at him. 'He's ter-
rible at guitar though—all paws.'

She was standing there, grinning at him
again while Hendrix wasted no time in saying hello by sniffing him closely, right in the
crotch area. Chris gently pushed the dog's
nose away and moved behind the surgery
table. He was keen to keep his distance from
the eager hound. Looking at the woman before him, who was dressed in every colour of
the rainbow and still beaming like an idiot,
he moved a little bit quicker. Hendrix's eyes
followed him, but he didn't move from his
owner's feet.

'So, what seems to be the issue with Hendrix today?'

'Oh, just the usual. He needs his jabs and
worming, of course; the shelter checked for
a microchip but nothing came up. He's prob-

ably an ill-thought-out Christmas present. These dogs get so big… I don't think people realise.' She patted Hendrix on the head, and he looked up at her with a goofy. adoring look on his face.

'So, you're adopting him?'

The woman laughed. 'Sorry, I don't think we've been introduced properly. I'm Susannah Harkin. I work with the local shelters. I lost my Labrador a few years ago, and I couldn't quite wrap my heart around getting another dog. I went to look round the shelter one tragically sad afternoon…' Her voice cracked, and the rest of her words didn't leave her mouth. They seemed to hang there, in the air, and Chris found himself wondering what they would have been. 'Anyway…' She seemed to shake herself mentally, and the smile was back. Chris almost squinted as he felt the brightness invade the room. 'Here I am. I foster some of the dogs that are a bit too much for kennels, work on a bit of house training, get them ready for their for-ever home.'

'Is there such a thing these days?'

'Such a thing as what?'

'A for-ever home,' Chris retorted. 'Our throwaway society seems to feel different.'

The woman looked a little thoughtful. A

second or two later, she bent to stroke behind Hendrix's ears and eyed the vet over Hendrix's head.

'Maybe, but you don't throw the baby out with the bath water. Not in Puddle Lake anyway. People do care. The way I see it, if I can help a few dogs get a better deal, then it's more than worth it. Bit of company around the house too.'

Chris found himself nodding despite himself. She did have a point—just thinking about going home chilled his blood. It was too quiet, devoid of life. He found himself sitting at home waiting for work to start, but then work started and his mood didn't improve.

'So, Hendrix here just needs the usual MOT. A bit of training, a good groom and he should be good to go.'

Hendrix looked up at Chris, a comical expression of horror on his features as though he could understand everything the pair of them were saying. Typical dog—they all loved the vets until they had some kind of treatment, and then the pooch soon wised up for the subsequent visits. Hendrix was looking at the door and Chris followed his gaze. Susannah was still staring at him when he realised he hadn't spoken for a full minute. In all honesty, he was with the dog. He wanted out of this room, right now. He snapped back into vet mode and pushed his own muddled thoughts aside. He was becoming a pro at it too.

'Okay, well, let's get him up on the table and see what's what.'

The scared Doberman, as though he had understood every word, suddenly pulled up on the lead Susannah was holding, her face registering the movement just a second too late. Hendrix, now fully aware of the impending doom that was coming his way, threw his whole body weight against the door, letting out a pitiful howl in the direction of the vet's waiting area.

'Woof—woof!' Hendrix was pulling at the lead with everything he had, trying to dig through the wood of the thick surgery room door with his overgrown claws. 'Woof! Woof! Woof!'

'Hendrix! Come…on…!' Susannah, knocked off balance by the terrified hound, ended up on the floor, partly beneath the dog, partly wrapped in his lead. She looked like a rainbow, her coloured clothing spreading out around her and Hendrix's brown chicken legs hopping all around her as the dog made a valiant but ultimately futile bid for freedom. 'Hendrix, please!

Cut me a break. I told you this was coming. We had a deal, buddy! I bought you a pup cup in good faith, damn you!'

The dog paused for a moment, looking Susannah in the eye and giving her a long lick up her cheek before returning to his frantic scrabbling and high-pitched whines of frustration and fear. Chris looked at the bright and scattered woman flailing on the floor, and at the dog, and sighed.

'Hendrix, stop.' He didn't shout it, but his deep controlled voice stopped both Hendrix and the woman beneath him in their tracks. The dog looked at him and slowly turned away from the door, standing on Susannah in the process; he then sat quietly at Chris's feet. 'Good boy.' He patted the dog once on the head, and then, looking at his surrogate owner sitting on the floor agog, Chris held out his other hand. She eyed it warily for a long moment, Hendrix seemingly in awe of the vet now and obediently waiting for the next instruction. She wiped her now muddy hand on her clothing and slowly put her hand in his. Her hand felt warm, and surprisingly soft to the touch. His jaw dropped a little, the shock of the contact enveloping his body. He hadn't held a woman's hand in what seemed like a lifetime. He slowly pulled her to her feet, his other hand reaching for hers as she come to a stop right in front of him.

She's quite pretty. Beautiful green eyes, with that red hair. Sea glass and fire.

She slowly pulled her hands from his.

'Thanks. Sorry about him too.'

He grabbed his stethoscope from his desk and came to kneel by the startled hound.

'Not to worry. I think we've come to somewhat of an agreement. Hendrix, let's get this over with.'

Dr Jennings inspected Hendrix, noting things down on his computer screen as he went. Susannah watched him work his magic on the bedraggled canine, who was now allowing the vet to investigate his undercarriage without trying to rip his arm off.

'So, you're the new vet, then? Not some weirdo masquerading under his name?" He sounded nothing like the outgoing vet had described.

'Stating the obvious, since I currently have a thermometer in an awkward place.'

Hendrix's face was a picture, but Dr Jennings looked as if he were sucking on a lemon. Susannah pressed on undeterred.

'Settling in okay, then? Must be different

for you, from a big-city mega vet to this little corner of the world.'

'It was hardly a mega-vet. We only had six partners in total.'

'Well, our whole village has *one*. Trust me, to us that's a mega-vet. When we got Starbucks on the motorway exit everyone went nuts for weeks. We only had the tea shop in town before then. There was even a petition to get it closed down, but thankfully the caffeine seemed to fend off any real feuds. So, you liking it?'

'I've been a vet for a while now,' he rebuffed, his face stony. 'Hendrix is fine, and his jabs are now up to date.'

'I know that.' She ignored his attempt to shut the conversation down. 'I meant living and working here.'

What was this guy's problem? She was only trying to be nice. It was like trying to talk to the dogs at home. Hendrix had a better line in conversation than this sour-faced man. He was rather cute though, she noticed as he got to his feet and went back to his computer. He was tall, dark-haired, and would be handsome if he didn't scowl all the time. Dr Ingham had made a strange choice for his practice. Ezekiel Ingham was like Santa Claus compared to the tightly clenched man before her. She knew Ezekiel had been looking for a while, and the last time she'd been in to talk to him about her dream of an adoption drive, he'd been excited for his successor to arrive in order to give him some much-needed time off. He'd been a stalwart of the local community for years, but now his children were all flying the nest and raising chicks of their own, he was looking to slow down. From the way he'd spoken to her about Dr Jennings, it had seemed as if he was going to be a perfect fit. Now, as she watched him tut at the screen, banging at a couple of keys a little too hard, she couldn't really see what Ezekiel had been thinking.

'Are you having a bad day or something?'

He ignored her, his face lit up with the glare of the computer screen.

'Hello? Earth to Dr Jennings.'

'What?' He almost snapped his reply at her, and she felt herself frown for the first time that day. Even Hendrix hadn't annoyed her to nearly the same degree as the man standing in front of her. He finally turned to look at her, and she noted a touch of regret cross his features. 'Sorry, did you say something?'

'I asked if you were having a bad day.'

He frowned, his almost black brows forming a tight frame around his dark brown eyes.

'No worse than any other day.'

'And?'

'And what?'

'And is that good or bad?'

'It's just a day. It's a dull Wednesday afternoon, my clinic is full, and I got assaulted by a Doberman.' He looked at her, his face pulled into a sour expression.

'Well, a day is what you make it. I find that if you try to find the joy, it's there.'

She could tell from his expression that he thought she was some kind of 'Be Kind' hippie. Which she was, in many ways, but it still irked her.

'Not always. Are you having Hendrix fixed?'

Great, and now he was talking about dog testicles. He really didn't want to be spoken to, did he?

'Yes, please. I am hoping to get him rehomed as soon as his training is done.'

The vet said nothing, turning again to the screen.

'I can do the operation next week. Monday morning?'

She frowned, getting her diary up on her phone.

'I can't, I'm on shift that day. I can do Tuesday and Wednesday?'

He sighed heavily, squinting at the screen and tapping a few keys just that little bit harder than was required. Susannah and Hendrix were both watching him, and from Hendrix's unamused face, she could tell he wasn't impressed by the new vet's mood either.

'Tuesday I can fit him in first thing. That suit?'

Susannah nodded, making a note in her phone diary.

'Perfect, I'll be home to look after him then. So what's the verdict?'

'He's fine, a little underweight, but that should correct itself over time. He's quite healthy for a stray.'

'Oh, he wasn't a stray; he was surrendered to the local dog shelter anonymously.'

'Ah, the behavioural issues make more sense now.' His jaw flexed. 'I do hate how people think these animals are disposable.' He printed a quotation sheet off the computer, coming around the desk to give it to Susannah. As he passed the paper to her, he knelt down and gave Hendrix a rub behind the ears. To his credit, the hound for once took it in his stride, and gave the man a lick. He laughed, and Susannah saw the vet's demeanour change. His shoulders relaxed, his expression changed from a deep-seated scowl to show a handsome face, and his eyes now looked less like a shark's. The change in him surprised her.

What was wrong with him? It seemed like more than a bad day, but looking at him now, playing with Hendrix, it was hard to reconcile the two men.

'Do you have any pets?' she asked, suddenly interested to know more about him.

'No, sadly not. I never had the time before I moved.'

'And now?' she pressed.

He looked up at her then, Hendrix sitting with his tongue out, clearly loving the ear scratch that Dr Jennings was giving him. *Fickle,* she said to Hendrix in her head. He had been trying to bound out of the door a second ago, and now he was shamelessly leaning into the vet's touch. From the look on Dr Jennings's face, she realised that the thought of having his own pet had never occurred to him.

'Well, now I guess I have more time. I've never thought of it like that.' He gave Hendrix a last stroke and stood up straight. Susannah had to look up at him, given his tall stature, and she found herself looking at his body. Just for a sneaky second, before she caught herself. She wasn't here for any of that. She was here for the dogs. Which reminded her of the charity drive she desperately wanted to get up and running.

'So you might be in the market for a dog, then? Maybe you can get one at the charity drive.'

'Charity drive?'

Susannah's heart sank. She could tell it was the first he'd heard of it.

'Yeah, I did have an arrangement with your predecessor. We have a bit of a backlog with the rescue dogs in the area, and I'm a bit overstretched. Having a charity drive would be a great way of matching some with new owners and raise some funds too.' She had eight dogs at home, including the overexuberant Hendrix, and she was starting to feel a little stretched. Her job was emotionally and physically draining too, and although she only worked part time, it was still a lot. There was barely room for her in her own house, and it was getting costly. The shelters she worked with were amazing, but she tried to chip in with the costs when she could. Non-profit charities cut costs where they could, but the money still never seemed to stretch far enough.

'Right, and Dr Ingham agreed to this on my behalf, did he? He never mentioned it, and as he's away…'

He trailed off, standing there in silence. He was dismissing her! Susannah felt her hackles rise.

'Well, yes. He's away, but he did say that the practice would help. I was actually hoping to start the ball rolling today.'

His eyes were on the clock before she'd finished speaking.

'Well, I don't have the time today, I'm afraid. I have a patient waiting.'

'It won't take a minute. I just wanted to check you were on board. Perhaps arrange a proper meeting time, so we can discuss it in more detail. If we could have vet support, it would make a real difference.'

He made a kind of squeaking noise in his throat, as if he were being strangled.

'Well…er… I am new to the place, and my caseload is full. I really don't think—'

'Tuesday, then, you'll have the time. I can sign the consent paperwork beforehand.' She wasn't about to let this drop. He looked put out, but she smiled at him and turned to Hendrix. 'Right, you, home we go!' She turned to leave, the image of him staring at her open-mouthed etched into her memory.

This drive is going to be more of a task than I thought. I wish I were on a cruise. So I could beg the nice vet to come back and sort this sourpuss out.

He was going to say no, and she wasn't about to let him do it without a fight. Her house was packed to the rafters, and so were the shelters. They were having to turn dogs away now, sending them further afield. It broke her heart, and a man who acted like Ebenezer Dolittle Scrooge wasn't going to put a kink in her planning.

The door closed behind her, and she walked into Reception, Hendrix's lead pulling as he spied the main door. She gave him a look, and he sat down at her feet. The waiting room was quite full. Maybe Dr Jennings was just busy, tired even. She wasn't one to be down; it wasn't her way. That didn't mean she didn't struggle herself some days.

'Everything okay, Suze?' Cheryl asked her from behind the desk. 'You look like you've had a bad day.'

Cheryl's choice of words made her cackle with laughter.

'You could say that. It started well.' She nodded her head towards the door. 'I need to book in for Hendrix here.' She made a snipping movement with her fingers. She never liked to talk about it in front of the dogs. She felt a bit sorry for them really, but it was for the best. Less chance of any more unwanted puppies to rehome down the line and fewer health complications in later life. 'Tuesday first thing, please.'

Cheryl clicked on her keys, nodding along.

'All booked in. Sixty-five pounds for today on the account, okay?'

'Elvedon Shelter for this one, please.' She had accounts running at the vet's for the shelters she worked with; she was the dog whisperer in this little corner of the world, and it was easier than paying out and having to claim it back. She wasn't broke, but she wasn't flush either. She owned her house and land, and loved her job, but she still had to be careful to watch that she didn't spend all her money saving dogs. 'I'll see you Tuesday.'

She was about to put Hendrix in the car when Cheryl called her name. She was jogging across to her, a furtive look on her features.

'Sorry, did I forget something?'

Cheryl waved her away. 'No, no. I just wanted to catch you to ask something. What did you think of the new vet?'

Susannah wasn't one for slating people she had just met, but she did find it very hard to bite her tongue without ripping the whole thing off.

'Well, I think bad days are catching,' she said diplomatically. She hoisted Hendrix into the back of her car, waiting for him to settle down with a treat she'd lobbed in before carefully closing the boot. 'Why do you ask?'

Cheryl looked back at the practice before answering.

'It's just…he's been a little bit…'

Susannah saved her from speaking. 'Moody? Surly?'

Cheryl nodded in relief, her eye still on those front doors.

'You did notice, then. He's a nice bloke, but…the transition is a little tricky, especially when Ezekiel went away. He needed it though—I'm just not sure the locals are accepting it very well.'

'The charity drive is dead in the water now too,' she muttered, more thinking out loud. 'What's his problem?'

Cheryl, never one to gossip either, looked uncomfortable again. 'It wouldn't be for me to say, but…'

'But?' Susannah found that she really was interested in the answer. She leaned in, and, looking into the boot, she could see that Hendrix was regarding them both rather intently too. 'You know I won't say anything.'

'It's his wife…' Cheryl gave in. 'I think she left him or something. When he was talking to Ezekiel about the job a few months ago, I'm sure Ezekiel said he was married. No wife, no ring.' Cheryl bit her lip, obviously feeling very guilty about her admission. 'I think it's because of her. He never gets any calls, you know? Nothing personal. The closest he got was when we had a kitchen firm call him about something about his house. I think he's a bit lonely perhaps. I just hope he settles in soon.' She gave Susannah an odd look, and then it dawned on her. She knew why Cheryl had been so eager to talk to her. She wanted her help. The resulting groan from the very depths of her soul made Cheryl wince.

'I know but come on! You make everyone happy around here! And…and…'

'Need a hand, clutching at those straws?' Susannah's mouth twisted into a tease. 'I can't help on this one.' She looked back at Hendrix, who had now settled down in the back, as if butter wouldn't melt. 'I only just met the guy, and he didn't exactly roll out the red carpet. He shot down my charity drive and—'

'The charity drive, that's it!'

Cheryl jumped in the air like an overexcited meercat.

'That's what? He practically threw up when I mentioned the idea. He is not on board.'

'No, I know he's probably a bit reluctant...'

'A bit reluctant? He walks around like he could sweep the floor clean with every tight step he takes. He doesn't give a fig about the charity drive, and why would he?'

'He loves animals!'

Susannah rolled her eyes theatrically.

'Rather a given, with his job.'

'No, I mean he really loves animals. He's been berating the patients' owners since he got here for not looking after them properly. He's a bit of a stickler for animal care, and he shows real passion.'

Susannah couldn't help but frown. The guy Cheryl was describing didn't sound anything like the angry vet she had just had the displeasure of meeting. He was curious about Hendrix's background though. Maybe he did care, just a little. 'I don't know, I don't really have the time.'

'That's what the charity drive was about, wasn't it? Getting more dogs rehomed, enticing more foster carers. It will all help, right?'

Susannah soon felt very tired, leaning her head against the back window. Hendrix jumped up and tried to lick at her forehead through the glass.

'I'm not sure I'm the best person for this, Cheryl. Me and men...'

Cheryl patted her on the shoulder. 'I know, but this is just business. It won't do you any harm to get out of the house a bit more either.' Susannah was ready to cut her off, but then she thought of her last weekend off. She'd not left the house, other than to walk the dogs. Even that had been on her land. She'd done it in PJs and wellies. It was hardly packed with action. The closest thing she got to excitement these days was when her Amazon book orders came. Cheryl had a point, but she couldn't help but feel irked by it. Cheryl could tell, judging by her face. 'Please? For me?'

Susannah snorted. 'The last time you rang me and said that, I ended up with a three-legged dog.'

'Yeah, and he got you moving again! Come on, after Beau, you needed some company.'

And the rest, Susannah thought.

When Beau, her old Labrador dog, had passed away, she had been lost. That was true. Cheryl had thrown her a lifeline asking her to foster a dog for the practice, and it had gone from there. Company in her house, but she was still not sure how she would get on with Dr Jennings and his stunningly rude bedside manner.

'I'll give you that, but you will also remember that I do better with male dogs than with their human counterparts. I'm not sure I can help this time.' She was slowly edging to the driver door, but Cheryl was clearly torn between trying to rope her into her plan and heading back to work to keep the chaos caused by Dr Mardy to a minimum. Susannah half followed her, one eye on the surgery door.

'Just think about it, okay? For me? One little chat. Maybe take him out for a coffee.' The look on her face was all gentle smiles and begging eyes, but even with the help it would generate, not to mention making her life easier, her mind was still screaming at her not to get into bed with this man. Metaphorically speaking, of course. She couldn't really imagine any woman wanting that little slice of delight—well, not with his scowling demeanour, anyway. It would no doubt be rude and perfunctory, just like his dog bedside manner. She did wonder what was under his clothing though—she could still appreciate a good-looking man when she saw one. If he smiled, he would be rather attractive, she thought.

'I'll think about it,' she said eventually, but she saw Cheryl's shoulders sag. 'Come on, Chez, you know me and men.'

'I knew you and one man,' she said softly. 'You can't keep measuring all your experiences with the same yardstick.'

'Well, I've heard my ex called other things before, but never that.'

Cheryl laughed, and Susannah smiled. She loved making people happy—making them laugh, even. Even if it was as a result of poking fun at her marriage and the subsequent rather messy divorce. Still, that was in the past. She wasn't as affected by things as she once was, but Cheryl's comment did make her think. Did the people who were in her life really think that? Sure, he'd cheated on her, and treated her as second-best pretty much the day after the wedding—a whirlwind wedding at that. She'd been a fresh young nurse, and he'd been the powerful, commanding doctor. He'd wooed her, married her, and then promptly forgotten about her. She'd been the idiot who had fallen for it, but it had been first love. She'd never met anyone she cared about like him. He had tamed her free spirit, but then just assumed that she would take life, and his shenanigans, in her stride. It was a huge shock to them both that this simply wasn't true.

'I'm well shot. Happy as a lark.'

CHAPTER TWO

As SHE DROVE away from the surgery, Hendrix looking out of the window excitedly, Susannah thought over her encounter with Dr Jennings. She knew now why he had irked her so much. Oh, sure, his mood was sullen, and she didn't gel well with people who lived under a cloud, but it was more than that. He'd reminded her of *her* doctor. Commanding, a little bullish when it came to work, condescending even. *Handsome.* She mentally crossed that last one off the list in her head. Her husband had been handsome and look where that had led. The nurses she'd worked with had loved it, much to his delight and her disbelief. The thought of dealing with a man who made her feel like that reminded her of him; it drained her energy. Even Hendrix seemed a little subdued in the back. The pair of them travelled in silence, till she clicked open her electronic gates, and drove the car up the long drive to her house.

She loved Solitary Cottage. An odd name to be sure, and not really a cottage either. Not by traditional standards anyway. It was a huge place just for her really, but when she'd been reeling from her divorce, and wanting to leave her job in the city hospital where he reigned supreme, the local hospice in the little-known Yorkshire village she'd grown up in had been looking for a nurse. And when she'd first gone to the estate agent's, looking for a home to replace the one she'd shared with Duncan, Solitary Cottage had immediately caught her eye.

It wasn't just the name, of course, although that had screamed out to her when she'd first been told of the listing. It had been in a good state of repair, just a little unloved. It had only stood empty for three years, after the former occupants had aged and left for something more manageable. With their children living abroad, the house had been put up for sale, and eventually forgotten about. Too much of a fixer upper.

In those three years though, standing empty and forgotten, the few acres that came with the land had really come into their own. Now, as she let Hendrix out, free to roam the secure grounds, she opened her front door and was hit by a wave of nostalgia. The first time she'd got the key from the agent and driven up here, she had been met with resistance. Not from the neighbours, who were all quite happy behind their own fences and friendly from the off. From the house itself, it had seemed. Ivy had been growing through a crack in the window. The vines had slipped in, and eventually pushed through the rest of the glass to wind around the hallway. A pile of post wrapped in these vines had rendered the door firmly shut to visitors, and it had taken her a good twenty minutes to cut and rip and squeeze in through the door frame. She'd taken one look around the place and offered on it the same day.

She put her keys into the dish on the hall table, and, drawing breath, she went straight through the house, Hendrix in tow, heading to the back of the kitchen. Opening the back stable-design door, she walked out with Hendrix and closed the bottom half of the door off. Her back yard was more than a back yard, with the land that sprawled from her property, but it was welcoming. She felt safe here, even on her own out in the sticks. She liked that the place was a little out of the way in Puddle Lake.

She had divided the grounds into two sections: one for her to grow vegetables, read in, have a glass of wine in and sunbathe, the other for the dogs in her care. She had a row of heated plush kennels, a wash area, a separate kitchen and even a grooming room. She had made it her project over the years, with help and funding from charity events and the local council. Even now, sometimes it took her breath away at how much she had achieved since walking into this house, her old Lab in tow, and the ink on her divorce still fresh. It had been the start of something new. Which made her think, what was Dr Jennings here for anyway? The same reason? To live a quiet, easy life in this beautiful backwater? If it was a change of pace he was after, as he had alluded, then he didn't seem happy about it. Maybe he was regretting leaving his city life?

The wife thing was odd too, but she knew first-hand that saying *I do* wasn't a guarantee of a happy relationship that lasted for ever. Not every love could be like *The Notebook*, after all. Frogs and princes looked exactly the same with rose-tinted glasses. Experience took the blinkers off, but by then the damage was done. Maybe he was just dealing with stuff. Or not, as the case may be. She'd

turned into Nurse Dolittle after her failed relationship. If she hadn't had her rescue dogs
to fill the hole, maybe she wouldn't be as
sunny as she was now.

Opening the door to the run, to which
the dogs had access from their kennels, she
beamed as she was engulfed in a happy re-
union with sloppy tongues, waggy tails and
the sense that, in their world at least, she was
important. She wasn't second best. She won
first place in their hearts. And they in hers.
Although, she did wish she could share it
with someone, a man who saw her through
their puppy-dog eyes and vowed to put her
above all others. She sighed, the dream of a
man popping into her head once more. He
never had a face in her daydreams, and that
depressed her even more than the thought
that it would never happen. She wasn't even
dating, so it was hardly a surprise. She got
to work sorting the dogs out and tried to forget about her day.

'Cheryl, I do appreciate what you're saying,
but as the new owner—'

'As the new owner, I of course defer to
you. However, the clients are not happy.'

'The clients are the animals. How many
complaints have you had from them?'

Cheryl's head snapped back as she digested this.

'Well, none, of course. You're very good with the animals; I'm not disputing that.'

'So this conversation is over. Yes?'

'Yes. No!'

Cheryl puffed out air from her cheeks and put one hand on her hip. Chris resisted the urge to smirk. He was annoying her, and it gave him an evil thrill. Till Susannah's face popped into his mind. Her comments earlier on that day had got to him over the course of the day, and he felt a tinge of guilt for winding up his assistant. He didn't make a habit of abusing staff. It was something he disliked intensely. He pulled his face into an apologetic expression, showing that he was listening.

'The thing is, Dr Jennings, the clients are happy, but they don't pay the bills. Their owners do, and the level of complaints is getting a little much. I just wanted to address it, and I did have an idea.' She looked up at him then, getting into her stride now she had his ear. 'The charity drive with Susannah.'

Chris felt his gut sink into his boots. 'Oh, God. No.'

'Susannah needs the help. She's had such a lot of new dogs come in recently, and the shelters are full. She's overworked, and it's not cheap, what she does.'

'Is this her job?' He slapped himself mentally. Why did he need to know? He wasn't going to do it. Not a snowball's chance in hell. He was pretty sure they would annoy the heck out of each other. She was far too... happy.

'No, no. She works at the hospice; she's a nurse.'

Chris felt as if the blood were being sucked out of his body with a straw. He felt a little wobbly on his legs. 'The hospice? Really.' A thousand images assaulted his brain, but he turned his back on them all and plodded on. 'Well, if's she's so busy, she must have help from somewhere.'

'She doesn't. It's just her. Her house. She does everything for the dogs, and her patients. She needs a break. It's not been easy for her. She could employ someone part-time eventually, I suppose, but that's a way off. Especially without a cash injection.'

'You seem to know a lot about her—are you friends?'

'Yes, I guess we are now. She came to us at a difficult time, losing her old dog, but then she fostered one for us.' From the look on her face, Chris surmised that she'd had something to do with that as well. He would have to watch his back. 'It grew from there, but now she needs this charity event to come off. And you need a little bit of goodwill in this village. People talk around here, you know. There are other veterinarian surgeries too, and although they're a little further afield I would hate for us to lose out on any clients.'

Chris frowned. 'Am I really that bad?'

'One client, who shall remain nameless, called you a bullish oaf. Another one said that Dr Spock was friendlier than you, and just yesterday I overheard a conversation in the post office. Your name was mentioned, and it wasn't a recommendation.'

Chris winced, and she fell silent.

'I'm sorry for that. Who called me a bullish oaf?'

'Client confidentiality, I'm afraid. The charity drive could be the perfect way to turn it around. Show the villagers your other side.' She cocked her head to one side. 'You do have one, yes?'

'Have what?' he retorted, much less grumpily than he felt. Her words stung him, but it was a sting of shame. He had been numb for a while now, but he'd obviously overstepped far more than he cared to.

'A good side.'

He nodded his head, just once. 'I have. Somewhere, in the back.' He pointed to his head, and Cheryl laughed.

'I thought so. Will you think about it?'

'I will. I'll discuss it with her when she comes back with Hendrix.'

Somewhat satisfied, Cheryl left him to it after that. She was his ally with the patients, and he didn't want to alienate her or make her job harder than it was. The news that Susannah worked as a hospice nurse had levelled him when he'd first heard. Now he could see it. She was so happy, so colourful. Maybe that was why she was able to do what she did. She obviously had a caring heart. He knew he couldn't do it. He never wanted to set foot in one of those places again. He could still remember the smells, the sounds, the staff. The nights of watching his wife sleep, till her final slumber. It was like another lifetime, but he knew every detail, as if the memories had plugged themselves into his skin, pumping constant reminders into his thoughts, his senses. All it took was the scent of her perfume on a pet owner in the clinic and his memories zapped into life and his movements grew shaky and stilted.

They'd not been perfect, Chris and his wife. They'd had to work at their marriage, like everyone else, but broadly they'd been happy. They'd had their lives sorted, together. They hadn't been waiting for the next step, or lacking something. They hadn't talked about their future, or about what might come next. They'd married in a low-key affair, after an easy and short engagement. They had met, and just clicked. Like a key into a lock. No flash of passion, just a recognition that they were good together, happy in each other's company. Their sex life had been good, comfortable, and not lacking in passion. They'd both loved their careers, yet still made time for each other. They'd brushed in and out of each other's lives, had a great big circle of boozy friends to go out with on a weekend. They had been busy living their lives, working away, or staying overnight at their jobs when it was needed.

When the cancer had come for her, he'd realised just how much she'd meant to him, and they'd spent every last moment together. And he'd grown angrier by the day. Not at her, not at the cancer. At himself, he supposed. At them both. They'd had such a busy life together that when they had nothing but each other, and endless treatments, and time off work, they'd stalled. He'd been there, a constant by her side, but he'd realised, with an

overwhelming clarity, that they had needed
more than each other. They hadn't known
each other as well as he'd thought, and as
they'd sat there, day after day, waiting for
some hail Mary that never came, they had
known that they never really would. He'd
buried a wife he didn't really know, and his
anger was complete. He'd wasted time, not
fully loving the woman he was married to,
and now she was a memory.

His life was over too. Not in a devastated
Cathy and Heathcliff way. He was grief-
stricken, of course, desperately missing his
wife and crying over her pain at the end. Life
was cruel, and impossible for those left behind. His life was over because he didn't fit
into it any more. He was the widower now,
in a high-flying, high-living bunch of friends
who were all either dating serially or were
married off. He was something that they
didn't understand now. His house was empty,
his calendar the same. Work didn't quite hold
the same appeal. He found himself wondering why he'd taken so much on, always working when he hadn't really needed to. They
hadn't had any children to provide for; they
had been more than comfortable. Now that
he didn't have any reason to rush home, he
realised just how much he wanted to. Wanted

to get home early and meet his wife in the hallway. Strip her bare and say hello properly, take his time. He would have cherished her more, learned more about her, and never put work before her. Ever.

It always taunted him. Hindsight was an honest and rather bleak realisation, and it kept hitting him over and over.

When he got home to his empty house later that night, the house his legal-eagle wife would never have wanted to live in, he pondered his own madness once more. He'd changed his life, slowed down, moved across the country and set up in a small village, cashing in his ticket for the fast lane once and for all. He had all the time in the world now, but he still had nothing but work. So he worked, and studied at home, keeping up to date with practices and techniques, but he knew it was a distraction. He'd created the kind of life he thought he should have now, but he only felt as if he'd got angrier. After all, what was the point? He was still alone, with his work and his house, and his money. Sure, he was comfortably off, but that was because he never spent a penny. Now that he wasn't even going out and enjoying his free time, the only thing increasing was his bank balance. His mood had dropped lower than a snake's belly, and now he was a mean boss to boot. His clients and neighbours hated him, and he felt as though he was being hogtied into helping the last woman in the village he would ever want to spend any time with. Mrs Sunshine-on-a-Stick.

The more he thought about Susannah Harkin, the more his mood soured. It just categorically could not happen. He would rather face the wrath of the likes of Mrs Chan before he would agree to working with that woman. The surgery would put up flyers, and that would have to be enough. A nice gesture of support. He shuddered, thinking of how happy the flyers would be. He had visions of his windows looking as if a rainbow had vomited on them, and his resolution to stay out of the charity-drive business hardened. He'd just have to be nicer to his clients, and find something to change his dark moods when he felt the familiar flickers of frustration and hopelessness erupting within him.

CHAPTER THREE

'I'LL GIVE YOU anything you want if you do what I say. Please. I'm begging you.'

Susannah tried her best alluring look, keeping her gaze fixed on the big, dark eyes in front of her. 'You know it's going to happen. I know it's going to happen. Let's just do it, get it out of the way. I can't bear this, us pussyfooting around each other.'

The eyes stared back, silent and unreadable. Susannah groaned in frustration, her head dropping onto her knees. She was sprawled outside the surgery doors, half hanging out of the bush into which Hendrix had just pulled her. He was sitting in the bush next to her, his lead loose, his flappy ears drooped low with his head.

'You won't feel a thing. My uncle Alan had the same operation, and he was fine in a day or so. Bit sore, but it's for the best. We don't want lots of little Hendrixes running around, do we now?' Ever vocal, Hendrix made a disagreeing growling sound beside her, and darted back into the bush when they heard footsteps approach.

'Everything okay?'

'Oh, great, it's Mr Sunshine.' She said this under her breath, but when she peeked out from behind a clump of leaves, she could tell he'd heard her.

'I prefer Chris most days. You are aware that you're late for your appointment, yes?'

Susannah clenched her teeth. She didn't have access to her watch right now, given that she was hanging like tinsel in the bush, but she knew she couldn't be more than a minute or two late.

'Technically, I am on the premises. And arrived perfectly on time.'

'Yes, but the council tends to object when I castrate animals in the car park. Do you need help?'

Of course I don't, not from you. I would rather take up residence in the bush than ask you for help, but I'm pretty sure that the long lead is unravelled and wrapped around my feet.

'I might. Is Cheryl inside?'

She could have been wrong, but she thought

she heard him laugh. It surprised her that he knew how.

'No, Cheryl went on break right after she informed me of your arrival. She sent me to get you.'

Cheryl, I wish you a crappy break. I hope your biscuit drops into your tea, you meddling little witch. Maybe she had more than Earl Grey in her teabags. Eye of newt, perhaps.

'Right. Brenda, then.'

Given that Brenda was the cleaner, and only worked when the surgery was shut, she didn't expect an answer.

'Am I really that bad? I am going to be operating on your dog today. I do prefer my customers not to be terrified of me before I pick up a scalpel. Come on.'

He helped extricate her and Hendrix from the bush, half tangling himself up with her at one point when Hendrix realised he'd been scuppered. He made a last dash for freedom just as Susannah found her feet, but her legs were suddenly lassoed to his rather lithe trouser-clad limbs, and Hendrix was very vocal all the way through. She heard Chris curse as he reached down and gave a good strong tug on the lead to free them both up. He put his hand out, and she took it while she steadied herself. Chris pressed the release button on the retractable lead, and it sprang taut. Hendrix came to a stop and sat at his feet.

'Oh, now you co-operate!' She turned back to Chris. 'Thank you.'

'Training going well, then?'

Susannah bristled. 'It's a work in progress. Any hot-blooded male would fear today's procedure.'

Heading into the surgery room, Hendrix subdued but somehow calmed by Chris, she gave him a pet and Chris gave him to the nurse on duty to take into the back, ready for surgery. When the door closed, they both stood in silence.

'Do look after him—he's a good boy really. He just needs a bit of discipline.'

'He'll be fine, don't worry. I'll make sure to call you when he's in recovery.' He paused for a moment. 'Nice to have a day off work though, eh. Are you working later in the week?'

Susannah answered him without even questioning why.

'Not till the weekend. I have another possible foster dog to look at over at one of the shelters. They just got a stray in from the local RSPCA inspector.'

'Right.'

'So let me know if you know anyone wanting a dog. I think I'll have to bring this one home too, to be honest. Bit of a sad stray.'

'Mm-hmm. Shame.'

He didn't say anything else, so she really had no idea how to broach the subject of the charity drive. Normally, she could slip anything into the conversation. Given that she didn't even want to have the conversation in the first place, she was feeling more than a bit put out.

'Yes, it is a shame. Lots more like him too. Me and all the fosterers I know are packed to the rafters. The shelters are cracking under the weight of all those unwanted, unloved little doggies.'

'It is a problem.'

'Yes, but a problem that we could fix. Right?'

'Wrong. There will never be a home for every dog, given that things don't change. It's the system that's broken.'

'I agree with you there, but there is another thing we could do. Other than going all Targaryen and breaking the wheel. We could do the charity drive, for example.'

'I did already say that I would put the posters up. Didn't Cheryl tell you?'

'She did. We need more than that though,

and Dr Ingham did say that the practice would help.'

'And I plan to uphold that.'

'We need more than posters. We need people to help, real support. If we could get the surgery there, offering advice, meeting the dogs, it would really help.'

'We have a busy practice.'

'It's planned for a Sunday. When the practice is closed.'

His eyebrow rose.

'I am on call.'

'You also have cover. It's just a day.'

'Of unpaid work, yes. On my day off. I might have plans.'

'Unpaid, but those brand-new dog owners will need a vet, and who better than the one they met on the day?' She'd thought of that one herself, hoping that the prospect of new clients might just give him the push he needed. 'Think of all the brownie points you'd score with the locals too. Puddle Lakers are big animal lovers.' Cheryl had told her about the complaints. Mrs Chan was telling all and sundry that he was a haughty fat-cat-shamer. It wasn't the best look for the only vet in the village, especially given that the practice relied on the villagers as much as they did on the practice.

'You've got a point there,' he admitted with a peevish look to his features.

'Exactly, and it's only one day! You can do whatever you were going to do another day. What were you going to do?' Silence. 'Well, you don't have to tell me if you don't want to, but—'

'I don't really want to, to be honest, and now I have surgery to perform.'

Susannah took one look at his haughty face and something inside the colourful, upbeat woman she was snapped. Just a little, a crumbled corner perhaps, but the damage was there. He was thoroughly ticking her off now. She narrowed her eyes at him, giving him her best steely glare, and he mirrored it right back.

So annoying. He looks quite sexy now.

She focused on her glare, and not his penetrating gaze.

'Well, I guess there's no point in taking up any more of your time, then, is there?' She gave him a final look up and down, as if to sear her dislike to his stupidly arrogant and rather hot body. 'I'll let you get back to your patients. No doubt they're all missing your wonderful bedside manner.'

She half yanked her bag out of the room in her hurry to get away from him. She was halfway across the reception area when she realised that every animal and adult in the waiting room had been listening to the entire exchange. They all jumped guiltily when she looked in their direction, many pairs of eyes swiftly avoiding her gaze.

'Bye, Cheryl,' she called, and then she was out of there. She heard the door swish closed and open again behind her, but it wasn't Cheryl's eyes she met when she turned to see who'd followed her. He started to walk over, but she didn't let him open his mouth.

'What is your problem, exactly?' She rounded on him as soon as he neared her.

'I don't have a problem. I just can't help, and I don't appreciate the disruption to my surgery either.' Following the thumb jab he aimed behind him, she could see the blinds at the surgery windows moving. At one point a little black dog snout poked through but was swiftly pulled back through the gap. 'I have enough on, being new to the place.'

He crossed his arms, bringing her attention back, and she found the move insanely haughty. He was so arrogant! The flicker of attraction was doused out. She could almost hear the sizzle as the fire was extinguished.

'I apologise for the scene, but you're so frustrating! You *won't* help, more like. Not can't. You've been like a bear with a sore head since I met you, and I know I'm not the first villager you've annoyed!'

'Ha!' he scoffed loudly. 'You've managed to deduce my entire character after a couple of short meetings, have you? The jungle drums of the village been playing my sodding tune, have they? Well done, Agatha Christie!' Mrs Gallagher walked past them, her Schnauzer, Herbert, in tow. Neither of them had noticed her coming up the road, nor seen the flickering of the blinds in the surgery waiting room.

'Morning,' Mrs Gallagher trilled out to them both. 'Nice day, isn't it?'

'Lovely, yes,' Chris managed to stumble out.

'Yes, lovely,' Susannah replied, continuing to wave and grin like a robot at Disneyland. Chris nodded distractedly at her, both of them standing there awkwardly waving until she reached the surgery doors and went inside. From the corner of her eye, she was pretty sure she saw Cheryl's arms yank the pair of them through the doors. Chris hadn't noticed a thing. He was too busy tearing a strip off her. 'You see, this is the problem with these villages. People are too…'

'Nice? Friendly?' She spat the words at him as if they were bullets. 'Caring?'

'No.' He stuck his bottom lip out as a toddler who had been denied ice cream might. 'Nosy. Cheerful.' He levelled that word right at her. The way he said it, the way he locked onto her eyes… The bullet word he fired hit her right between the eyebrows and incensed her.

Who the hell did this misery-guts think he was, dissing her village?

'Well!' She folded and unfolded her arms wildly. 'It doesn't take a genius to spot a newcomer. Voldemort has more warmth than you!'

He unfolded his arms and followed her as she got closer to her car, keys in hand. 'Oh, so my mood is your business too now, as well as what I do on my day off? What's *your* problem?'

'*My* problem!' She gasped, leaning in closer and brandishing her key bunch at him. 'I don't have a problem. I'm just trying to do my job!'

'Oh, your job, how holy of you! It's not even your real job!'

How the hell did he know that? God, he was annoying! She had never wanted to slap someone other than her ex before, but her palm was tingling at the prospect.

'And? You have two vocations in life, do you not? Being a vet, and being a curmudgeonly old fart to boot! What are you, forty? My nana has more crack than you!'

'What *are* you talking about?' His hands slammed onto the car bonnet as she reached the other side, and she banged hers right back on the other side, mirroring him. They were circling the car bonnet now, leaning in with their clenched fists and getting right into each other's faces as they bickered. 'I don't have two vocations; I'm happy to just do my job and be left the hell alone. I'm not trying to be Mary sodding Poppins, like you! Swooping in, trying to save everyone. Give me a break and join the real world!'

'The real world! What would you know about the real world? You hide behind your table in there, with your foul moods and your scowling bulldog face. You do know the village thinks you're hard-faced, don't you?'

'I don't care what the villagers think!'

'You will when they all head to the surgery in town, and you have no one to bellow at. The charity drive would help us both.' They were both nearly screaming at each other now, the air heated and thick. 'You're just too thick or too stubborn to see it. Look after Hendrix.' She gave him a final glare, telling him in no uncertain terms that she was trusting him with one of her dogs, and she wasn't a bit happy about it. 'That *is* your job, after all. Even if you do hate the world, don't take it out on him. No wonder you're alone, when you act like this!'

'Oh, really?' He folded his arms as she got into the driver's seat, stomping round to her side door and leaning into her window space like an annoyingly sexy traffic warden. She hated herself for noticing how cute he looked when he was mad. He tapped on the window, and the moment was gone. As she wound her window down, she considered winding it back up and catching his tie in the process, but then decided against it. Dragging the vet behind her car, annoying as he was, wouldn't be a great look. Besides, he had Hendrix to operate on. She could plot his demise another day. She could hear him chuntering away, but the words were cut off till she had wound down the window.

'What did you say? Sorry, I had my window shut. Never heard a thing.'

Given that he'd been ranting like a mime against her closed window, she knew she'd missed the highlights but the satisfaction she got from seeing his impotent rage was a balm to her stressed soul.

'I said,' he retorted, his face a picture, 'that I might be alone, but some of us are happier that way. You obviously are. Despite being an annoying busybody.'

'I am not a busybody, and you set the bar for annoying!' She went to wind her window up again, narrowly missing his face. Through the gap in the glass, he got the last word in. 'I just think that the villagers and their animals deserve more than the Grinch in vet form. You suck!'

'Yeah, well so do—' The rest of his comeback was muffled by the window, and she cupped her ear dramatically, motioning with her fingers that she couldn't hear him. He gave her a finger of his own as she pulled away, and she gasped in shock. All she saw before she focused on her driving was him laughing at her shock.

God, I could just smash his smug little face in!

'Horrible man!' she shouted as she pulled out of the car park, smacking the steering wheel for good measure. 'I mean, the gall of him! I am *not* Mary Poppins!' She ranted to herself half the way home, and silently seethed for the rest.

It wasn't till a few hours later that she got her nerves to stop feeling so jangly. She wasn't easily irked, but Christopher Jennings was the type of man she detested. Haughty, work-driven, rude and selfish. He epitomised everything she couldn't stand. And had been married to, once upon a time. The charity drive would just have to go ahead without him. After today, she wanted nothing more to do with Dr Moody Pants. He could keep his help, and his ruddy finger gestures. His laughing face would be in her nightmares for the rest of the week.

'Hateful man!' she shouted out into the ether. She saw to the dogs, made herself a cup of tea, and headed out into the garden with them. A bit of violent weeding would be just the thing to quell her rage towards a certain veterinarian from hell.

Chris checked Hendrix's vitals for the third time, and then cursed himself for allowing the argument and Susannah's barbs to get to him. The finger gesture had definitely been beneath him, but she got under his skin so much his fingers had tingled with the sudden urge to flip her off. He felt a twinge of shame at his actions now, which was only heightened by the fact that the whole surgery had obviously seen the free show. He'd lost himself in his work for the rest of the morning, switching his brain off and focusing on the medicine.

Hendrix's surgery had gone smoothly. The hound was now stable and awake, and looking more than a little fed up in his large cone collar. Chris had no appointments for the moment, so he sat down on a little stool they used in the back area, next to Hendrix's open cage. Hendrix moved a little bit closer to him, and Chris gave him a nose rub.

'She's quite mean, your foster mum. Did you hear what she said to me?'

Hendrix let out a low groan. Chris nodded at him.

'Exactly. You get it, right? I'm a good vet. I do care.'

Another low moan.

'And I'm not alone. I'm just…'

He trailed off. He couldn't even lie to the dog. She had a point. He had been a bit of an ogre. To everyone. No one had had the gall to say anything to him though, back home or here. Being called on it by her, of all people, was more than a little annoying. She didn't know him at all, yet here she was, making him feel bad for merely living his life.

'The point I'm trying to make, Hendrix, is

that your "mother" is the one in the wrong here. I would help, of course, but I don't have the time.' Her comment about what he did on his day off came back to haunt him. She did have a point there. In all honesty, other than work at the surgery, he was home, rattling round his empty place. *She didn't have to know that though.* It wasn't any of her damn business, for a start. People like her only ever saw the good, never the bad, and that happy-clappy way of thinking just wasn't something he could do. What was the point? People were horrible to each other all the time, and they survived. A bit of dog-fat-shaming and abruptness didn't suddenly make him Voldemort.

He knew it was more than that; he knew it was that her job made him feel sick to his stomach. The fact that she could be so happy to boot, well, it just made no sense to him. He'd spent his fair share of time in a hospice, and he couldn't imagine working in one. Selfish though that might make him, it didn't mean that he didn't care. Looking at Hendrix, he sighed heavily. The dog mirrored him with a sigh of his own, and reached out his long tongue to give his hand a lick. Chris gave him a pet, and leaned in close.

'You're not a bad dog really, are you? I

hope you do find a home, no matter what people might think. No one should be lonely. You have a kip now; I'll ring Cruella for you.'

He chuckled at his own joke as he went to look on Hendrix's file. All of the dog's known history was there, which wasn't much. Just a rudimentary profile really, along with flags for challenging behaviour. As he looked up Susannah's number, his gaze fell on the details of the shelter, and something else popped into his head. Looking back at Hendrix, who was now snoozing in his quarters, he had an idea.

CHAPTER FOUR

SUSANNAH WAS IN no mood to hear from Chris, but she wanted to know about Hendrix. She let the call from the surgery number go to voicemail, listening as soon as the message popped up.

'Er...hi...huh-huh...' There was the sound of throat-clearing. 'It's Dr Jennings...er... Chris here. Just to let you know that Hendrix's surgery was very successful, and he will be ready to collect when you're ready. I...er...hope the visit today went well.'

Susannah's eyes widened. He sounded quite...*nice* for a change. Genial, even. Asking about the new rescue dog she had told him about too.

Strange. Maybe he's given himself a personality transplant at the same time he removed Hendrix's crown jewels?

She was in the car park of the vet's already, the timing of his call not lost on her. She had a very scrawny and matted dog in the back, and Cheryl had told her by text to bring her straight up. She didn't even have room in her kennels for the poor little dog, whose breed she wasn't even sure of at this point, due to the muck and the leaves matted in its fur. The poor thing was wrapped in a blanket, shaking like a leaf. She'd need a lot of care, and Susannah already had Hendrix on her plate. She was getting to the point where she would have to say no to taking a dog in, and she didn't relish the thought. It left her cold.

The dog burrito she was carrying sniffed the air of the surgery waiting room and retreated further into her cover. Cheryl took one look at the bundle in her arms and came around the desk.

'Come straight through to the back,' she instructed, smiling at the people in the waiting room to allay their shocked faces. Susannah saw them, and felt a fresh surge of anger at the people who had neglected the poor animal in her hands. Cheryl pushed through the door, and led Susannah straight to the room they kept in the back for longer consultations. Susannah's phone chirruped in her pocket, and Cheryl gently took the dog from her.

'You get that; I'll get this little one registered,' Cheryl said.

It was her colleague from the Elvedon Shelter. They normally called to check on their dogs when operations were involved.

'Hey, Adam, everything okay?'

Adam said his hellos and got to business. Chris came out of one of the consultation rooms, his gaze falling on hers. She gave him her best scowl as she listened to Adam's excited ramblings. Chris's lips twitched, and then he smiled at her before heading into the room.

'Ugh,' she said out loud.

'What? Are you not happy about it?' Adam's confused tones filled her ear.

'No, sorry, Adam. I was distracted for a minute.' *By an oaf.* 'What did you say about Hendrix?'

When she went back into the room, the little bitch on the table was now lying on top of her blanket while Chris inspected her. Susannah stood at the back, and Cheryl was nowhere to be seen. Probably in Reception dealing with the other patients.

'She's got a strong heart. Lungs are good.' Chris took a wipe and cleaned the poor dog's eye area, inspecting them and her teeth. 'She has a few teeth that are too far gone. I would put her at about eight years of age, so the oral care hasn't been maintained.' He checked every inch of her, tutting occasionally when he noticed something he didn't like. 'She has fleas, which we can treat here. Angie will bathe and treat her.' He began clipping her nails, but the dog had other ideas. She emitted a sudden high-pitched scream that didn't let up and got higher and higher the more he tried. The poor thing suddenly tried to take a leap off the table, and they both jumped to catch her. She ended up half in his arms, and half in Susannah's.

'God, she's a livewire, isn't she?'

Chris nodded, a broad smile across his face. 'Certainly is. She'll be fine. She just needs a little care, and time to gain a healthier weight. Are you taking her home, or back to the shelter?' Susannah sighed, the tiredness taking her over. She was back at work all weekend, and she didn't quite know how she was going to pull it off.

'My house, I think. I have asked on the WhatsApp group chat for a foster, but everyone is already up against it.'

'WhatsApp group?' he asked, a jovial tone in his voice. 'What do you call it, Fosterers Assemble?'

She looked at him, confused. 'What?'

He stammered a little, trying to go for the

nails again but the dog was not having any of it.

'Like the Avengers? Can you do me a favour, please? Hold her? The nurse is busy.'

Susannah stepped forward, cradling the dog in her arms and comforting her while Chris swiftly treated her. 'There, all better.' He lowered her back down onto the blanket. 'She's a beautiful-looking dog.' He leaned in and scratched her behind the ears. The little dog, now discovered to be a very shaggy Pomeranian, leaned into his touch. Running his wand over the scruff of her neck, he sighed. 'No ID; she's not chipped.' Susannah's heart sank, as it always did, but it wasn't entirely unexpected. 'We'll get her cleaned up and treated for fleas, de-worm her and get her some food. I'd like to keep her in overnight, for observation. She's a bit dehydrated for my liking. I'd like to put her on a drip.'

'Thank you,' Susannah replied, earnestly this time. She was glad of the extra night to get organised.

'Do you think she has a shot of being re-homed?'

Susannah could see the dog shaking on the table, and she knew that it would be a hard sell. 'Well, her age isn't great for rehoming, and with her appearance and issues, it might be a while. I have work this weekend too; I'm not sure how much help I can be. With her and Hendrix and the others, it's all been a bit much of late.' She realised he was looking at her intently, and she brushed her melancholy away. 'Sorry, just a bad day. Preceded by a really hard few months. Hendrix has a home, though—the shelter came through, so that's a silver lining!' She said it a little too shrilly, and he noticed.

He didn't say anything. He nodded, taking the dog wordlessly into his arms. 'Give me a second. I'll just settle her in.' He paused. 'Do you have a name? For her records?'

Susannah always named the dogs, the ones that didn't come in with one anyway. She never changed the name of the animals; they had been through enough, without an identity crisis to boot.

'I…er… I…' She scrambled in her head for a name, but he cut her off.

'Don't worry about it.' He looked down at the little dog, who looked right back at him with such sorrowful eyes. 'We'll take care of her. Give me a minute.'

He headed out of the back door towards the quarters, and she could hear him communicating what needed to be done to Angie. Angie was the best veterinary nurse around,

and she was more animal herself than human.
Susannah could hear her talking to the dog,
telling her everything was going to be okay.
Susannah sagged against the table.

Would it be all right? All the time she
took these animals in, found them homes,
but there were always more. More puppies,
more owners who were ill-educated and un-
prepared for what owning a dog really meant.
More family issues that led to the heartbreaking and unavoidable decision to rehome their
fur babies. There were so many reasons, so
many animals.

Her hospice job was her main passion, but
she knew that her 'hobby' had turned into
much more, and it was running away from
her. She thought of Hendrix, cheered by the
fact that the Doberman was sorted at least.
The new owner had even elected to take him
home from the vet's, and deal with the recovery. She felt relieved, but she knew the space
was filled already by the bundle of fur she'd
just brought in.

The door opened, and she didn't bother
to look up. Her head felt nice in her hands,
heavy. It was all she could do to stand up,
she was so tired.

'Susannah?'

She met Chris's eyes, and straightened

herself up, smoothing her rumpled clothing down. She smelled of the dog now, and she knew from the stinging in her own eyes that it wasn't exactly pleasant. 'Yes?'

He looked her up and down, and she bristled under his gaze.

'I know I look a mess.' She gestured to herself. 'Is she okay? How's Hendrix?'

'They're both fine. Angie is bathing Loki as we speak. She'll get the matted hair clipped off, then we can see what we're really looking at. Hendrix is a little tender, but he's happy enough. Wolfed his food down. He's got an appetite.'

Susannah snorted with laughter. 'You're not kidding. I hope his new owner is prepared.'

'I'm sure they'll manage.'

'Yeah, the shelter said that they'll collect him themselves. A bit unusual, to be honest, with him healing. I'm a bit worried, but they said he'll be in good hands.' Her own hands were wringing together now, her bag strap getting twisted between her fingers.

'I'm sure he will be well cared for. Would you like to see him before you go?'

Susannah blinked rapidly at him.

'Susannah? You okay?'

'Yeah, sorry.' She frowned, feeling her

whole forehead crease down to her eyelids. 'No, I'm not sorry. We don't exactly get on. What's with the nice act?'

His lips pursed tightly. 'It's not an act. I'm not a complete jerk.'

'Not complete, no.' This was supposed to have been said under her breath, but it reverberated around the room. 'I would like to see him.'

He nodded, his arm sweeping towards the door. 'Ladies first.'

They headed straight to Hendrix's quarters, and Susannah's heart swelled. He looked so happy to see her, his tail wagging, his talkative voice in overdrive.

'Okay, it's okay! Gentle, Hen. Gentle.'

She sat down on the floor in front of the cage, not wanting Hendrix to get up and rip his delicate stitches. His cone was off now, but he was sporting a rather cute T-shirt.

'For his healing,' Chris offered. 'I do hate those cones. Some dogs do better without; Hendrix wasn't a fan.'

'Fireman Sam though?' she asked, clocking the decal on his T-shirt. Chris blushed.

'I buy them from charity shops, to keep in stock. It was either that or Angelina Ballerina.'

'Good choice.' She laughed, imagining

Hendrix in such a shirt. 'That would only add insult to injury.'

'Exactly. More street cred with this one.'

They laughed again, and Hendrix was wagging his tail with gusto now. *He's quite funny,* she thought absently. She focused on Hendrix, who was still making noise for her to give him more attention. She leaned in, looking at his big brown eyes. She hated this bit. She always tried not to get attached, but Hendrix was one of a kind. She'd even considered keeping him, but she knew it wouldn't be fair or practical. He needed a lot of attention, as well as love. She had her neighbours and the other shelter staff to help, but he needed to be top dog somewhere. He deserved the best. She leaned in and dropped a kiss on his nose through the bars.

'I'll miss you. My skirting boards won't, but that's another story. I hope your new home is everything you want it to be, my darling.' She felt her lip start to wobble and pushed a hot tear away before Chris saw it. She was being silly. He wasn't dying; he had a new home! It was the best-case scenario for him, but the shock of it happening so fast, coupled with the month she'd been having… well, it was enough to make even the most chipper of people feel a little bit emotional.

'I wish I could have had you longer,' she whispered, wiping her eyes and standing up again. 'Okay, so if the little one is staying here, I might as well get off. Will you let me know how she is in the morning?'

Chris nodded, looking at her in a way she couldn't quite read.

'No problem. Hendrix will be fine—they both will.'

She smiled at him, before remembering their earlier quarrel. 'Sorry about before. What I said was a bit harsh.'

He studied her, his eyes narrowing. 'But you don't regret it.'

Foiled. She had attempted to smooth things over without dredging things up again, but this man was as stubborn as she was, clearly. 'No, I don't. Not all of it.'

There it was again. That raised brow.

She steeled herself for another heated exchange.

'I'm sorry for my part too. I know what you're up against. I should have been a little less…well, surly. I'm not really one for getting involved in things. Not lately, anyway.'

'I get it. It's just, in my line of work, and with the dogs I care for, you tend to get mad when people moan about their lot in life.'

His jaw clenched, and she stopped talking.

'When did I ever moan about my lot?' he spat back, his whole demeanour changing.

'I didn't mean it like that.'

'Yes, you did. I haven't known you long, but I know that you say what you mean. I still have scars from the last tongue-lashing. You know nothing about me.'

'Neither do you know anything about me, but you still dismissed me as some kind of hippie weirdo. Judgemental much, or just plain mean?'

His meaty hand banged against his chest.

'Me! Judgemental? Mean I might give you, but I am not judgemental.'

'Oh, come off it, I only told you what everyone was thinking. Life's too short to be such a Dennis downer all the time. If you could see my patients, you'd soon understand.'

His face dropped, and his eyes went glassy. With rage, or something else, she didn't know. He looked as if his whole body was vibrating.

'I have seen patients like yours. Many of them, in fact, and it's not something I'd like to relive any time soon.' He looked straight at her, and she wanted to cut her own tongue out.

'I didn't know.' Her voice was devoid of

anger, softer. 'I am really sorry to hear that. Someone close?'

'I don't want to talk about it, if you don't mind,' he retorted, a little kinder this time. 'It's not something I like to talk about.' Susannah watched the utterly grim expression he had and decided not to press further. The pieces were clicking together in her head, and they added up to one word.

Widower.

The mystery of his wife, his sullen outlook.

He's grieving. And not very well, by the looks of things.

She'd never picked up on the signs before, but now they were flashing at her. She'd made a right dog's dinner of this, and she felt awful for her part in that.

'I understand. Well, I'll be off, then. Thank you for looking after them.' She lifted her hand to give him a pat on the arm but left it hanging awkwardly instead. It would have been too much. For them both. She was still stung by their argument. She understood him a little better though, and that unnerved her a little.

She went to check in with Cheryl.

'The dog's all booked in now, another one for the Bluebell. Chris named her Loki.'

Cheryl nodded, making a note on her computer. 'Aww, I like that. A nice strong name. Thanks, love. I hate it when they don't have a name, let alone a history. Poor thing. Good news about Hendrix though, eh?'

Susannah felt a pang. It reminded her that she wasn't leaving Hendrix here for the night, she was leaving him for ever. It made her grey mood even worse.

'Yes, losing his testicles and gaining a forever home, all in one day! He's had quite the adventure. I'll really miss him,' she admitted. 'I'm happy for him, of course.'

'You have plenty of wagging tails to keep you occupied,' Cheryl cheered, but she gave her a searching look. 'Are you okay?'

'Yeah, fine, you know me.' She went to leave, but what Cheryl said next stopped her in her size eights.

'At least you'll still get to see him. Old Frosty Pants says he's going to bring him here.'

'What?' Susannah's head whipped round so fast her neck clicked in protest.

'He's— He's not—' She jabbed her finger towards the room she'd just exited. 'He's never adopted Hendrix!' She jabbed at the door again, the keys in her hand flying around like spikes on a tumbling hedgehog.

She bounced on the spot, glaring at Cheryl till she answered. Cheryl was up and out of her chair, looking at her as if she were currently talking to a demon. 'Tell me.' She half growled, and Cheryl's eyes went wide.

'Well, he has a soft side. Who knew?' She shrugged, and Susannah resisted the urge to scream.

Sitting in her car, she gave herself a minute to collect her thoughts.

Well, she had tried to put her key into the ignition, but her hands were shaking so much that she was still no nearer to sliding it in than she had been the first twenty times. She pressed the lock button on the dashboard, locking herself in, and pushed her seat button to full tilt. Lying flatter now, her seat belt off, she closed her eyes and crossed her hands over her chest. It was a little trick she'd learned just before she filed for divorce—and the week after she'd lost her temper and almost thrown a brick through her ex's Porsche window. He had been parked outside a restaurant at the time, eating inside with one of her former friends from the hospital. It was probably the one and only time in her life when she had felt such pure hot rage. The realisation had shocked her. She'd known then that the feelings would only get stronger, and the residual anger needed to burn out in a healthier way. So she'd learned techniques to quieten her mind, to zen her out, and to stop her from kicking people who annoyed her, like the vet, as a reflex. She was feeling murderous again at the mere thought of him.

Back to the technique. Slow your breathing. Everything is okay. You can't change everything. You can't save everyone.

It was a weird little mantra, to be sure, but it worked for her every time. Even on the truly dark days. She always got through it. When she thought about it, she was happy. She was glad for Hendrix. Chris did calm him; she'd seen it herself. Even she didn't have that bond with him. It was as though Hendrix had chosen him, she realised. That was the moment every person in her position hoped for. That look of love and 'it's you' between them, and she knew that they would be fine. She'd missed the signs with the two of them, because he had acted like Mr Darcy on arrogance hormones, and that had riled her from the off.

Hendrix had seen it though, and she laughed. A small little chirrup that burst through from her lungs and didn't stop. She laughed hysterically, so confused and amused by the unexpected news that she just had to laugh. Maybe Hendrix would be great for him—some company to laugh at, something living to tend to. It was pretty perfect, and she realised that her interaction with the vet was meant to be. She'd helped him without even meaning to. With a bit of luck, that crazy, loveable dog might just be the thing to thaw out Mr Frosty. Which meant her charity drive might happen after all. Especially if she let slip how much of a 'hero' Dr Chris Jennings was. She could see the headlines in the weekly parish news now. This was going to be great.

'Mr Frosty Pants and Hendrix,' she said out loud, and then she laughed even more. By the time she got home, greeted by happy faces and wagging tails, she was positively jovial.

'Hello, my babies! I have so much to tell you...'

'For God's sake, will you just shut up?'

Chris rolled over onto his back, pulling one of his pillows over his face and yelling curse words into it till he felt better. Another resounding howl sang out from downstairs, and Chris threw the pillow across the room. It hit a canvas on the wall opposite, knocking it to the floor with a thud.

'Okay, foul beast,' he growled, pulling the covers off himself with force and stomping to the stairs. 'I'm up! What's the problem now?'

Entering the kitchen, something hard, yet also crunchy, jabbed into his bare feet. Yelping in pain and confusion, he flicked the light on. A raw piece of penne pasta was stuck to his foot, as well as a fair few crushed cornflakes, and something sticky.

'Oh, no, please!' He turned to the open cabinet, noting the dripping honey bottle, complete with teeth marks. There were cereal containers lying on the floor open, half of their contents crushed into dust. Hendrix was sitting in his basket, covered in honey and cornflakes and looking as though butter wouldn't melt. In his little T-shirt, he looked like a naughty toddler coming down from a sugar high.

'Hendrix!' Hendrix lowered his head, groaning loudly. 'Don't you try to get out of this. I know it was you.' Another low moan. 'I mean it now, no back talk.' Hendrix lay on his side in his basket, looking at Chris out of the corner of his eye. 'You are in trouble. Shower time. Upstairs now, but wait—'

The second Chris opened the kitchen door, meaning to turn around and explain that he would get a sheet to cover him, Hendrix was up and out of the door, cornflakes and goo flying behind him. Chris took one look at his cream-carpeted stairs, and tried to reason with the hound.

'Hendrix, stay still. Your stitches. They could tear or get infected. It means more time on my table, buddy, and neither of us wants that, eh?' He held the sheet like a matador would to a bull, his steps slow. Hendrix had bolted straight to the top of the staircase, which he had decorated in what could only be described as a whitewashed colour scheme. It was all whites and creams, a nice bright colour to let the light in. Chris hated to feel trapped indoors, but right now he wished he had embraced some goth chic, or something nice and dark to hide the damage. As if Hendrix knew what he was thinking, his head started to move from side to side. Chris's steps were getting faster as he tried to corner the dog and carry him into the fully tiled and easy-to-clean bathroom. The whole room slowed down, and Chris took one step closer. Hendrix's head moved faster, and he shook himself out in the corner of the room.

'Hendrix, no!' Chris tried to dive onto the recovering monster, to stop the contents of his kitchen cupboards being spread any further. Hendrix saw him coming and jumped right over Chris's back, bouncing straight into the bedroom, where he promptly sat down on the bed. Chris hit his head on the wall, ending up in a heap in the corner, only just avoiding the stairs. His leg was wrapped in the sheet, and he had a cornflake stuck to the end of his nose. And from the smell of it, it wasn't honey that held it in place. It was dog slobber. He looked across at Hendrix, who was licking the food off his paws and leaving a Doberman-sized print on the bed cover.

'Right,' Chris said, sighing heavily. He plucked off the cornflake, threw the sheet into the laundry bin, and looked right at his new charge.

'I'm going to get a good stiff whisky, and then we are going to try this again.'

He headed down the stairs, crunching through the cornflakes and Lord knew what else on the floor. He headed to the liquor cabinet, and when he couldn't see a glass, he shrugged and took a deep gulp from the bottle.

He waited a minute or two, and then shook his head angrily and brought his phone out of his pocket.

'Cheryl? Yes, it's Chris. No, everything's

fine. Sorry for calling a little late, but I wondered…did the er…shelter have any care advice for Hendrix?'

'Care advice?' Cheryl checked, her voice tinged with confusion and amusement. 'Er no, nothing but the usual on diet and exercise. We don't know much about him. Susannah deals with all that; she knows what to do. Is there a problem?'

'No, no, all fine. Sorry to have bothered you, Cheryl.' He ended the call, sighing heavily.

A second later, Cheryl sent a text message.

Call the dog whisperer. Be nice

She'd put Susannah's number at the bottom.

'Be nice,' he muttered, tutting. 'I *am* nice. Someone needs to tell Cruella to be a bit friendlier, if you ask me.' He took another deep burning swig of the liquor, and, after weighing up his options, he picked the phone up again with a huff. Dialling a number, he held his breath.

'Hello?' The tone was more confused than friendly.

'Er…hi.' He tried to speak again, but he

realised he didn't know what to say. Heavens, this woman!

'Was that all you wanted?' she asked, an amused tone creeping in. 'To say hello in the middle of the night? What's wrong, did you miss me at the surgery?' Sarcasm was there too.

'No, I...just a second.' He pulled the phone away from his ear and took another swig. 'Look, I hate this more than you do, but I need your help, please. I'm out of my depth here. I'm desperate, to be honest.'

The line was quiet, but he could hear the television in the background.

'Hendrix making himself at home, is he? Say goodbye to your skirting boards.'

'Oh, it's worse than that.'

'Oh, that bad, eh? Do you want me, or Mary Poppins? I'm sure she could turn her brolly in your direction if you asked nicely enough. Goodnight.'

'Wait! Okay, I'm a jerk, all right?'

'Sorry, what did you say? The TV's a bit loud.'

'I said I'm sorry.'

'And you're a what?'

'A jerk. A big jerk. I am desperate, Susannah. Would I have rung you otherwise?'

He didn't go as far as telling her Cheryl had told him to.

'Okay, you've grovelled enough, I suppose,' she replied, a happy tone in her voice. 'Need anything bringing?'

He was so surprised by her response that he didn't filter his reply.

'Yes. A bottle of whisky wouldn't go amiss.'

'On my way,' she replied, sounding very amused indeed.

'You rang?' she quipped when he answered the door, a once-white towel in his hands.

'Oh, thank God you came. He's running around in the bedroom now. I've had to shut him in to get the door.'

She didn't need to ask what was wrong. She could see the paw prints and battle scars from the doorway. She held aloft the bottle of good whisky from her home stash.

'Oh, you are an angel!' He ushered her in, keeping his distance.

'I would offer to take my shoes off, but…'

'Don't. I stood on a piece of raw pasta in the kitchen, and it felt like a skewer. You ready for this?'

'Bathing a dog?' she asked dumbly, somewhat enjoying the night's events. There was definitely more than one side to this man.

She found she rather liked him like this. 'Of course! Easy-peasy.'

Three hours, half a bottle of dog shampoo, and several meaty-flavoured bribes later, the house and Hendrix were as clean as they were going to be. The offender in question was now farting and snoring in his dog basket, which was lined with one of Chris's best bath sheets. Susannah and Chris had deposited him there wrapped in it and had not had the energy to get off the couch since. Chris had gone to get the whisky bottle at one point, and the two of them were sitting there, passing it between each other like bootleggers after a rough day at sea.

'I knew Hendrix was hard work, but that was something else.'

Susannah nodded, pointing her finger in the direction of his kitchen.

'Lockable cupboard catches on everything in my cottage. You have to treat them like toddlers. But smarter.' There was a slight slur to her words as she said it, and she hiccupped. 'Eyes in the back of your head.'

'I think next time I'll just move,' he deadpanned back. Susannah giggled, straightening herself up and getting ready to stand.

'I need to go. I'm on shift for the next week. Need my beauty sleep.'

'You're not driving, surely?'

Susannah shook her head. 'No, I'll call a taxi. Okay if I get my car in the morning?'

'How about I pick you up and drive you back here in the morning? I don't have surgery till later—we're having the new computer system installed at work.'

'Bet Cheryl will love that.' Susannah thought of her annoying receptionist friend and couldn't help but smile. She would love it, but she would never give Chris the satisfaction of knowing how much she'd wanted the surgery to modernise. She was still very loyal to Dr Ingham, and Susannah loved that about her, but neither of them had been about to ask him about it. His way had worked for many years, and he was an excellent vet in his own right. 'You sure you don't mind?'

'Well, I did drag you over here and ply you with drink; it's the least I can do.'

'The very least,' she mused, feeling her tired bones relax into the overstuffed couch they were sharing. 'I still smell of wet dog and honey.'

He chuckled beside her, holding aloft the bottle and looking at her questioningly.

'Go on, then, before I call a taxi.'

He passed her the bottle, his fingers brushing against hers on the glass surface.

'Why don't you come to see me at work, and see where we want to hold the charity drive?' She was lubricated by the whisky and, given that she had just helped him out of a huge mess, he did owe her. 'Come on!' She ignored his groans and choruses of, 'Oh, no, not this again.'

'Just one afternoon—you don't even have to stay long. I could just take you round the grounds, show you what I had in mind.'

'It's not necessary, really. I said I would help.'

'With posters, yes, but you know we need more than that. Seeing the hospice, and the staff, you will realise just what we're trying to achieve. Both sets of charities are so underfunded, it's a joke.'

She stopped talking the minute she looked at him. All easy traces of the man before her were gone. He abruptly stood up and stomped out of the room.

Oh, nice one, Susannah, she said to herself. *Way to overstep.*

He came bounding back into the room seconds later, thrusting a framed picture into her hands before he sat down again and focused his stare on the wall in front of them.

'My wife, Karen,' he offered as she looked at the frame in her hand. It was a wedding photo. Chris with an attractive blonde woman on his arm. They were both smiling at the camera. She looked every inch the doctor's wife. Elegant, well put together. Happy. 'She died in a hospice. She had tumours.' He swallowed, his jaw clenching and unclenching. 'It wasn't expected. Or quick.'

Having her suspicions proved didn't make Susannah feel any better.

'I'm sorry. I didn't mean to push.'

He waved her away with a shake of his hand.

'I get what you're doing, but I just can't go to one of those places. I get it, but I can't… Why are you holding the drive there? To split the profits?'

Susannah nodded. 'The dog drive will help the shelters, and they will be fundraising on the day. The hospice staff run stalls too, and they have an army of volunteers who all bake, sew and make things for the hospice to sell. Them having the gardens, with all the space…it just makes sense. The dogs will pull far more crowds in, and it will cut the running costs down for everyone.'

'Bringing your two worlds together, I guess.' He didn't look entirely happy with the statement, and Susannah knew he wasn't going to help. 'I get that.' He swallowed hard and reached for his mobile phone. 'I'll call you a taxi.'

She got up off the couch and gathered her things. Hendrix was still in his basket snoring, so she leaned in and dropped a whisky-smelling kiss on his snout.

'Enjoy your new home, mate,' she whispered to him. Looking across at Chris, who was watching her as he spoke to the cab company, she smiled at him. 'Look after each other.'

She thought she saw Chris smile at that, but he finished the call and was tidying up before she could blink. She followed him into the kitchen with a couple of empty plates from the sandwiches he'd whipped up earlier. She put the plates in the sink, but he wasn't in the kitchen. The back door was open, the light spilling out onto the lawn. It was a grand house, one of the best in the village. Dr Ingham had lived there for many years, raising his family in that house, like many other vets before him. It was an unspoken rule that once the departing vet wanted to retire, he would sell the house along with the practice—a way of ensuring that Puddle Lake always had a vet in residence. The house was a stone's throw from the surgery, and central in the village.

The lawn was huge, looking inky black in the dim light reflected from the windows of the house. It tapered right down to the few acres of land that came with the property, and wrapped around the house. It was gorgeous. It reminded her of her own land: peaceful, out of the way. In the dead of the night, she did her best thinking. Her best worrying too. She wondered what Chris did, when he was alone here. Did he feel it, as she did? Probably not. She stood in the doorway, lost in thought, and jumped when Chris spoke beside her.

'I have all this land.'

'I know,' she murmured. 'It's a lovely place. I've always loved walking the dogs round here.'

'Have the charity drive here,' he said suddenly, as if he would change his mind if he didn't say the words quickly. 'Have everyone come here.' He pointed off into the distance, where the field was empty, the bottom having a thick treeline that denoted the boundary of the neighbouring farm. They could just see the edge of the trees in shadow in the pitch-black night before them. 'I know you can't see it now, but there would be the space. You could have a marquee there, under the trees.

The dog show could be in the field, and I have plenty of parking. His long drive had grass on either side. She could see it suddenly, all there. The stalls, the dogs, her friends from the hospice running their family-friendly games and selling their wares. It would be perfect here, but she didn't want to speak yet. Chris was looking at her now. 'So, what do you think?'

'We'd have to bring the patients who can be transported here, so they don't miss out, but I guess we wouldn't have to be so quiet here. Will you help? On the day?'

'I'll be here,' he offered, his eyes the only thing she could make out clearly on his face. 'I'll do what I can, but it has to be here, and I don't want people knowing why.'

Susannah reached out her hand, and Chris shook it.

'It's a done deal,' she said happily.

'Yes,' he quipped, 'I think I just have been.'

The taxi beeped at the front of the house and he waved her off from his front step.

'It's not that funny.'

'Oh, I think it's hilarious.' Roz's laughter was as wild as always. Whenever Rosalind Ormsby found something funny, it was as if the joy had to burst from her, and it was quite infectious. She was sitting doing her charting in a quiet minute on the night shift. A quiet night was a good night; it meant everyone was settled.

It meant that she could catch up with her colleague too. Not everything was discussed at handover, and Susannah sometimes felt out of the loop when she'd had a few days off—how the patients were, and their families, and the shenanigans of the staff on their days off.

'I bet he was rueing the day that he ever signed his name on those adoption papers.'

'By the look on his face, I could tell it was pretty bad. It worked out well enough in the end though.'

It had been nice, sitting outside with him. Oddly comfortable.

Roz snorted and gave her a shove across the table with her elbow.

'That was it? You drank together, and then he just waved you off? How come he offered his land so easily? I thought you said he was some kind of Scrooge about it? Wasn't it awkward when you went back for the car?'

'No, I woke up really early, so I just got a taxi up there.'

'Chicken.'

'I am not! I put a note through this door explaining why the car was gone. You know me—once I'm up, I'm up. Rodney doesn't care for alarms.' Rodney, her rooster, was a bit of a warbler of a morning, but the truth was she'd been reading in bed when he'd made his first cock-a-doodle-doo. She looked around her, trying to avoid Roz's mutterings of being too independent and missing opportunities. The hospice nurses' office was as bright and cheerful as the rest of the place. In here, one wall was filled with photos and cards, well wishes and little keepsakes sent in thanks. She hadn't told Roz the story about Chris and his late wife, Karen; she had kept her promise. It wasn't her news to share anyway. She knew better than to add this to the idle gossip around the village.

'Ha. Rather ironic given that you're a total chicken. Fancy blaming the rooster. So that was it? He's just in now? I thought he was dead against it. Last time we spoke you were chuntering about turning him into a poster.'

Susannah sucked her breath in through clenched teeth. 'I know, but that was before. He *was* dead against it,' she said vaguely, 'but I think Hendrix changed his mind.' She did believe that her furry friend had made it a little easier to win him over. 'He's a good owner, you know. Hendrix seems really happy with him.'

That wasn't a lie; every day since that night she'd seen the pair of them walking around the village when she was on her way to or from work—Hendrix bounding around, Chris laughing as he threw the ball. It was normally very early, before the surgery and her shift started. She had started to look for him on her drive to and from work, and she was always so confused by what she saw. He was laughing, smiling. He looked happy. She felt a flicker of something whenever she tried to assess it in her mind. The only conclusion she could come up with was that she reminded him too much of his wife, with the job she did. There was nothing she could do about that, but she could abide by his wishes and not spread his personal struggles around the village. His wife wasn't her patient, but her duty of care still applied. If she had nursed her herself, she would not have discussed anything with outsiders.

'They make the oddest pairing but, looking at them together, it's nice to see.'

'Another one less to worry about, eh?' Roz signed the bottom of the sheet she was working on, depositing it into the in-tray. 'Speaking of which, when are we going to get this show on the road?'

'I have a meeting with him and Cheryl tomorrow morning. If I can stay awake long enough.'

She was coming off the back of a set of night shifts, which meant that her body clock was more than a little skewed. She'd booked the meeting for half eight that morning, not even thinking about the fact she would usually just be getting home to sort out the dogs before heading to bed herself.

'Eager beaver as always. You do so much for everyone—you need to remember to have some fun too.' Roz's eyes were on her, the black frames of her glasses making her look like a stern librarian.

'Telling me off again? I have fun.'

'Really? When?'

'Well, I took the dogs—'

'No, without the dogs. I'm talking about fun with other adults who can talk back.'

'We had that meal the other month! You were there! That was fun.'

'That was Sandra's retirement party, and she's teetotal. We were home by half eight!'

'So?'

'So, hardly living it large, were we? Did you ring that bloke?'

'The bloke with the crazy moustache who gave me his number on the back of a betting slip?' Susannah checked sarcastically. 'Oh, yeah, I slid right into his DMs. What a dish.'

Roz laughed, but she was like a terrier with a chew toy. 'Fair enough—he was a bit dodgy.'

'He looked like an e-fit from a nineteen-eighties crime photo. I've taken lumps off patients that were more attractive.'

'They're not all like that though, come on! Get on one of those dating apps, get yourself out there.'

'No, thanks. I live in a country cottage on my own.'

'So?'

'So I don't fancy getting murdered and my dogs eating me, thanks. Far too scary to risk.'

Roz guffawed with laughter. Helen, one of the nurses, popped her head around the door.

'Mrs Sutcliffe's family are here, Roz.' Roz nodded, getting up on her feet in an instant. She nodded at Helen. 'I'm just coming.' She looked at Helen again, and her eyes scrunched up.

'Oh, God,' Susannah said.

Helen, who was watching Roz eye her

warily, looked at Susannah. 'What? What's wrong with Roz?'

'Helen,' Roz declared, right before she put her face on and headed to do her job, 'show her your app. I'll make sure the floor is covered.'

She closed the door behind her and left the two women to talk. Half an hour later, Susannah left the office. The second she was out of sight, she deleted the dating app her mate had shoehorned onto her phone. Her friends meant well, but she wasn't about to put her heart out there to be trampled on again. Sure, Helen had met her now fiancé through the app she'd raved about, but still. That was one in a million, surely? She'd read enough bad stories to put her off dating full stop. Online was just too much right now. If ever, being honest. She watched the app uninstall and breathed a sigh of relief.

The fun barbs from Roz had stung though. She thought back to the last few events she'd been to, and she had to admit that they were all work trips, and things to do with work or the dogs in general. She hadn't been on a date in for ever, and the thought of lying naked next to a man had her reaching for the latest romance novel instead. She had to admit, her reading style had got a little more flirtatious, to say the least, but a woman had needs. It was just that she had been so hurt the last time, so broken, she didn't think she could do that again. She didn't have the emotional energy, or the sticky tape. She was whole now. She had her work, and her dogs, and her lovely little smallholding. She had friends, and even she and Chris had forged a sort of alliance. A weak one, but he smiled when he saw her now. He had a nice smile. She wouldn't dare to tell him of course; she just smiled back and carried on being herself. He still gave the odd eyeroll—normally at her brightly coloured outfit of the day—but she had been in and out of the vet's enough times to feel comfortable going. The clients seemed a bit happier too.

She headed along the corridor, calling into Derek's room. He was here on respite, and he had fallen asleep with the television on. She left the lamp on, tucking him in a little better, and turned off the television. She liked the night shift, and the peace it often brought her when it was like this. She thought about Chris then and tried to see the place she worked in through his eyes.

When people thought of hospices, they thought of cancer, or death. She knew that, and often it did mean that to the people coming in through the doors. It meant a step had been taken, and often those steps could not be retraced. She understood that; she'd held many hands, shed many tears, in private at home, or with her nurse colleagues in the break room. Some of the bleakest times in her professional life had been spent in that room, she and her colleagues holding it together for their patients and then later crumbling on each other. She knew that they were perceived to be like hospitals, but there was so much more than that to the work that went on.

She could hear Derek snoring softly, and she headed along the corridors, checking the rooms as she went. Chris categorically disliked her job and her workplace, but she knew enough about grief to realise that he was bottling up his emotions. Thinking about the dating app she'd just booted out of her phone, she knew he wasn't the only one. She thought of her meddling colleagues, the best women she knew with the kindest and largest of hearts. Just being around them might be enough to help her make that next move.

By the time she'd done her rounds, she had her plan in hand. She would help the hospice, the kennels, and Chris. It would do her some good too and distract her from the dating scene. Or lack of it. Expanding both of their social circles wouldn't be a bad thing, after all.

As she went to answer a call button, she was already looking forward to getting everything planned.

CHAPTER FIVE

'YOUR HOUSE?'

'Yes,' Chris said patiently, addressing his surgery team. Cheryl and the two veterinary nurses, Angie and Keeley, were both sitting in the staffroom looking across the table at him with faces agog. 'My house. Well, the gardens really. I will have St John's Ambulance there, portable toilets, the whole nine yards. The local pub will probably not mind people using the toilets either, given the extra custom it will bring. So that's the facilities covered. I know you all have contacts in the community, so do feel free to let them know what we're planning. And to contact Susannah Harkin. She should be here soon to talk to you all.'

He looked at his watch. He knew she'd been on a night shift. He felt a sudden flash of worry at the thought of her driving when tired. The woman never stopped. She made the Duracell bunny look like a monochrome sloth. She wasn't quite late yet, but he knew she'd finished her shift some time ago. He'd somehow along the way worked out her shift pattern, and he felt oddly comforted, thinking of her out there. She was his friend of sorts, he guessed. They clashed, sure, but he was finding it harder to be so melancholy with her in his life.

'So Susannah's in charge?' Cheryl pressed, a wry little smile across her face. Chris raised a brow.

'When isn't she?' The staff all laughed in response, and it gave him the push he needed. 'It's no secret that I wasn't exactly on board with this, but circumstances have caused me to have a rethink.' He looked across at Hendrix, who was currently on his back getting his tummy tickled. 'I know I haven't been the easiest person to work for since I arrived.' None of them said anything, which made him cringe on the inside. 'I just wanted to say that I am happy to be working with you all, so if you could bear with me a little longer, I promise we will get this place working well again, just like Dr Ingham wanted when he sold me the practice.'

'Hear, hear,' Cheryl said, lifting her coffee

mug to salute him. 'Come on, ladies, cuppas up. Three cheers for Dr Jennings!'

The ladies all lifted their teas and Hendrix bounded around their feet, joining in with his own little vocal tribute. Chris blushed right down to his shoes, shuffling awkwardly from foot to foot.

'Okay, okay. Thank you very much. Till Susannah gets here, let's get opened up and get on with the day then, eh?'

The staff all started chatting amongst themselves, Cheryl heading off to open the main surgery with Hendrix in tow. He usually sat behind the reception desk with her, and he had access to the gardens outside. He'd slotted in really well, and as Chris watched him get a fuss from Cheryl he realised that Hendrix had saved him too. Sure, he was a nightmare around the house. He went to the toilet as much as he ate, which was a lot, and Chris's pristine furniture was now covered in dog hair and teeth marks. There was a rose bush by the back door that would never recover from being used as a toilet, and his grass was now patchy in places from where Hendrix had hidden his many toys. Some of the pet-owning villagers had brought in presents when they'd somehow heard that Hen-

drix was now a permanent member of the
veterinary team.

Chris still had a full box out back, which
he was going to donate to Susannah and her
brood of furry charges. He owed her that
much. Bringing the dog into his life had
thawed out his customers for the better. He'd
seen a few of them on his dog-walking trav-
els. Some had even stopped to say hello. It
was a slow process, but he was finding that
he was a bit less of an ogre at work these
days. No more flipping off in the car park.
Thinking about Susannah's shocked expression behind the wheel made him smile despite himself.

He found he was eager to see her again,
but he couldn't for the life of him fathom
why. When she was around him, she annoyed
the heck out of him. Her enthusiasm was ex-
hausting, she dressed as if she was afraid of
the colour black, and she was just so…happy.
He'd never realised what a contrast he was
to her until they'd spent some time together.
The other night, at his house, it had been
different. She'd been calmer, and he hadn't
expected to see that side of her. Or that he
would like it. She was intriguing, and the
more he learned, the more he liked. It was
quite annoying, and if there was one thing

Chris hated, it was feeling as if things were happening out of his control.

'Roz, come on! Give me back my phone.'

'Are you kidding me?' Roz was swiping her finger across Susannah's phone, her face like thunder. 'You deleted it already? I knew it!'

'Roz, I tried, I really did!'

Roz's eyes pinned her to the spot over her glasses.

'Prove it. How many matches did you get?'

'What?'

'How many matches did you get?'

'I don't know. I've no idea what I'm doing on those things!'

'The match is when you both swipe right on a person's profile. Did you swipe on anyone?'

Susannah looked at her friend and considered what the best way to lie was. Roz shook her head, and Susannah rolled her eyes. Putting her hand out, she pouted back.

'Please, just give me the phone. I deleted it, okay?'

'How quickly?'

'As soon as I left the room.'

'Susie!'

They were preparing a room for a new client, making sure the relevant equipment was installed and that everything was ready to go upon their arrival. The patient incoming was Beryl Richards, who regularly came in to give her husband respite. Errol was devoted, of course, so keeping him away long enough to give him the rest he needed would be an issue, but Susannah was looking forward to seeing her patient.

The two of them always gave her hope. Their love for each other had got them through a car accident that had left Beryl with life-changing injuries, yet the two of them were the epitome of love's young dream. Beryl came here to give Errol a break, but she would always joke that it was a break for her too. She'd been a busy person before the accident, and that hadn't changed now; she was always helping with the fundraising. Errol had run his own timber-mill company at one time. He'd sold up for the most part, after the accident, but their sons still ran it together, and he was still known as the boss man.

The pair of them were so inspiring, and Susannah always filled her well of emotional caring just by being around them. It gave her hope for her own future. An abstract future, to be sure, but still. They were the couple she thought about when she considered dipping her toe back into the game of romance. Something that just worked, two people who put each other first, and rolled with the punches together. Tightening against the strain of life, rather than bending and shattering as her marriage did. She absently rubbed the space on her finger where her rings used to sit as she waited for Roz to stop talking about what a waste it was. How her friend should be living her life while she could.

'I know all that, Roz, you know I do! It doesn't make it any easier, does it? Dating apps just seem so cold. People use them for random meet-ups—how am I supposed to tell the difference? Plus, the first profile that came up made me want to throw my phone at the wall.' Roz raised a brow in curiosity. 'It was Neville.'

Roz emitted a little gasp.

'*Neville*, Neville?'

'Neville, Neville.'

'Well, well, well.' Roz looked quite impressed. Susannah shook her head.

'Don't even think about it, Roz.'

'Oh, come on.' Roz jabbed her jovially in the ribs with her elbow. 'Neville from up on Oak Farm is lovely! He's not been single that long either; Claire from the post office said he was considering going to Turkey for hair plugs. He used to have a nice head of hair, you know.' Roz fluffed the curtains so that they draped nicely in their matching tiebacks, staring wistfully out of the window onto the manicured gardens below. 'He was quite the dish back in school.'

'Yeah, when he was in short trousers, and he was always with Nancy Carrick anyway, remember? Since school!'

'Yeah, well, they're divorced now.' Roz leaned in, the way non-gossipy women did before they were about to gossip. 'Nancy's dating someone from Manchester. He comes in his flash car and takes her away for the weekend. I heard her say in the salon the other day that if she never smells horse muck again, it will be too soon.'

Susannah bunched her nose up. She didn't fancy Neville, but he was a lovely man. Having his wife up and leave him after twenty years had changed the man, and she just felt sorry for him now. He was trying to change himself for a woman he would never get back. She knew enough about heartbreak to realise that the dating apps and the hair plugs were just a way to appear as if he were moving on. Neville Rochester was a brokenhearted man, and she didn't see them hitting it off.

The truth was, she didn't see herself hitting it off with anyone. When she'd married, it had been for ever. When she'd realised that wasn't going to happen, she'd understood that she hadn't just lost a husband; she'd lost herself too. Her wardrobe had been muted down over the years, much like herself. She laughed a little too loud for his liking or wore something too eye-catching. She'd shaved off little pieces of herself, over time, for him. To fit into the world that had started as theirs and ended up being his. By the time he'd cheated on her, she hadn't known who the hell she was without him. She'd had to learn about who Susannah Harkin, née Danvers, was, and she wasn't about to offer her life up again for anything less than perfect. Since life and dating were far from perfect, it stood to reason that she would never find it.

'Ugh, that's awful. She was always a bit up herself at school. Poor Neville.'

'Exactly, poor Neville! On the dating app, looking for a nice woman to share his life with. He loves animals too!'

'He breeds lambs and has chickens—he's hardly David Attenborough. His dogs are all sheepdogs, and he refused to sign my anti-fox-hunting petition the other week—said he didn't want to ruffle any feathers. I don't need a man like that. What on earth would we talk about? I don't fancy him either!'

'Well, that's what the date's for! To find out, to take each other for a test drive. Some romances are slow burning. It's not always about ripping each other's togs off on the first date, is it?'

'He wears dungarees, Roz, not some silken Lothario shirt and sexy trousers. I'm a PJs and Jeep type of girl, and he's all tractor and double denim. Not compatible, and I don't want to date in the village! Too many people will know.'

'So? Everyone has a life, Susannah! Who gives a toss if people know? They'll figure it out one day.' Her eyes narrowed. 'Unless you were planning to just slip off into retirement with your bevvy of hounds…'

Susannah blushed. She hated being called out when she was being evasive. Roz always knew how to read her. It came easily after the years they'd spent working together, side by side. They knew just what was going on with each other, and it was extremely annoying at times. Times like this one.

'Well, what if I was planning to stay as I am? I'm doing okay: I have my own place, I can wire a plug and change my own tyres. I make my own money. Why bother looking? Come on, Roz, you're divorced. You get it. What's the point of doing all that again?'

'Because life is meant to be shared! Everything you just told me about is the boring stuff, Suze. You don't fall in love to split the gas bill or have someone to take the bins out.'

'Oh, I took the bins out when I was married.'

'Exactly. You can do everything on your own, sure, but why the hell would you want to?' Roz jabbed her finger towards the closed door. 'We see it here, every day. People wanting to live their lives, and be loved, and give love. Not everyone gets that. We see time being lost every day, Susie, and it's heartbreaking. When I got divorced, I was the same. You know I was.'

'I remember the gin and the sweatpants.'

'And the nights of crying on the phone to you, wondering what the hell was wrong with my life.'

'I remember.' Susannah nodded, making a sympathetic face to her long-time friend. 'It was rough.'

'We both had rough divorces, and, sure, I might think that my ex-husband is an amoeba on the backside of humanity now, but it doesn't mean I want to be alone for ever.'

'You're not alone though; you have all of us.'

Roz stared her down.

'I know, but it's not the same and you know it. Listen, I don't want to nag you—'

Susannah tried to cut into the conversation but Roz continued, shutting her down by talking louder over her.

'But I will! I'm happy dating Eric now, but I kissed a lot of frogs on that dating app first. It's life, Suze, and I'm not being funny, love, but you could use some.'

'I have a life!'

'Really?' The head tilt with the glasses again.

'Oh, come on, Roz, the bloody stern librarian look is getting on my wick now! I have a life.'

'I'm only "stern",' she bristled, throwing in a couple of hefty-looking air quotes, 'when I need to be. You sent me knitting patterns for dog blankets the other week.'

'And? I thought they might sell well. The knitting posse we have love new challenges.'

'The writing on them, Suze.'

'It's funny!'

'My mummy loves her doggies?' Roz was

aghast. 'It's one knitting needle in the brain away from *Live Love Laugh* blankets.'

'I've got a pattern for those too,' Susannah retorted, before biting her lip fiercely. 'Okay, point taken. I have let work take over a little bit, but I am happy as I am.' *Another lie. Wow, she was racking them up lately.* Roz harrumphed in response.

The two nurses headed to the next rooms, turning down beds, checking equipment as they went. Seeing to the patients and chatting to them, making sure that they were all happy, that rounds had gone smoothly and everything was on course. It ran well when the two of them were on the floor. They were two arms on the same body, they'd often joke. The team was so close-knit, they were never flappable even when under the greatest pressure. Unlike her current scattered panic at the thought of seeing another man naked. Or another man seeing her.

'I know you're happy, and that's great. You're complete; you don't need a man. I know all that.'

Susannah signed off a medication sheet after checking it over for the fifth time. They could natter, but they were always on the ball.

'I just think that having a man in your life would enhance it. You'd have someone to share it all with. The vet's quite nice, by all accounts. I'm hearing good things.'

'Oh, yeah, he adopts one dog and he's expecting his sainthood through the post.' Susannah always bit when he was mentioned. She pursed her lips. 'He's good with Hendrix though. He's not all bad, but I won't be dating him.'

'You don't know that. Anything can happen on all those late nights, poring over stall plans and best-in-show entries.'

'It's hardly going to be all *Dangerous Liaisons* and whispering by candlelight. We're meeting in the village hall, with the others.'

Roz pulled up her lip, Elvis style. 'That sounds like torture. Can't you bin the others off and change the venue?'

'Roz! It's a big event; we need people to man things, to sort everything out. We have to sort out a beer tent, food stalls, the whole lot. Chris apparently pulled his staff onto it, and now half the county wants to help. Which is great, but I feel like I might have a small stroke at times, and the dogs are all great at mine, but now I have a pregnant bitch. I wasn't expecting it—the intake vet at the shelter missed it. The foster I had lined up can't have a pregnant dog in the house because her husband's off work with a twisted disc.'

'Breathe.'

Susannah stopped talking and took a deep breath. 'You see? I don't even have time for a stroke, let alone a date.' She clamped her lips together when she replayed her words and put a finger up to shush Roz.

'I heard it. Don't say it. Let it go. You know what I meant. I can't date, Roz. I'd have to get dressed up, and shave, and…get naked! I can't get naked with a man, I just can't.'

Grant, a member of staff, came walking into the room at that exact moment, brandishing a set of forms on a clipboard. The two women looked at him, and he squeaked in panic.

'Leave the forms on the bed—I'll just be a minute,' Roz instructed him in a kindly way, and he sagged with relief, throwing the contents of his arms onto the bed and power walking his way out of the room. The door clicked shut behind him.

'Well, that was embarrassing. Very professional of me.'

'Oh, give over. Grant's heard a woman talk about sex before.'

'I wasn't talking about sex. I was talking

about being naked. I can't have sex if I don't want to take my knickers off, can I?'

Roz half pulled her out of the room and on with their duties.

'Listen, you never know. You don't want to get on the apps, the vet's nice. Single…'

'Wow, nice. Single. What's next? Has a pulse?'

'You'd be surprised. I dated a few zombies myself—you know, the obsessive types.'

Susannah nodded; she knew all too well. Work was the 'brains' her zombie ex-husband craved.

'He gets under your skin—I think that's worth exploring.' They headed to the office.

'If every man who got under my skin annoyed me, I'd be shagging half the neighbourhood.'

Grant was sitting in the easy chair, eating a yoghurt. He put it down and left wordlessly, putting his head down as he passed between the two women.

'Oh, dear God, I did it again.'

Roz's laughter exploded the second he closed the door. It took her a good three minutes to pull herself together, and that was even after Susannah had tried to kick her under the table, hitting the metal pole with her own toes instead.

'Damn you, I broke my toe!'

'Serves you right. Now go and ask the guy out, before I ask him out for you. Get him to look at your broken toe.'

'He's a vet!' She grimaced, pulling off her shoe and feeling relief when her toe wasn't splattered across the inside of her shoe. It felt more dramatic than it was. 'Not exactly his field.'

Roz clicked her ID into the computer, bringing up her email.

'You always had chicken feet—he'll have a look.'

Susannah's eyes narrowed.

Best mates always know what to say to wind you up. I don't dance like a chicken! I'm a swan. Especially after a couple of whiskies...

'Hey! My chicken feet stay in the best-friend vault, remember?'

Roz tapped away at her screen, but Susannah knew she was listening.

'I don't want to make it weird with the vet. He's not…'

'Hot? Single? An animal lover?'

'Available,' she ventured.

'Well, you won't know till you ask him.'

'No, Roz!'

Roz stood up suddenly, pulling her glasses

off and addressing her friend with a steely glare. Her eyes were sparkling with mirth, giving her away as always.

'Oh, yeah? You ask him out before the next village meeting thingy, or I email him the tiddly chicken video.'

Pure horror filled her.

'You wouldn't dare show him the tiddly chicken video. You promised to take that to the grave.'

'And I will, but this is for your own good.'

'How is showing any hot-blooded man the chicken video going to get me a boyfriend?'

'We'll see. I'll give you two weeks. Don't bother asking the girls to override me either—I'll fill them in. It's time to get your feet wet, Susannah Harkin. You are dipping those toes back into the dating pool whether you like it or not.'

Susannah ground her teeth like a petulant toddler. Roz was unmoved.

'You're a rubbish friend, you know that.'

Roz laughed again. 'Oh, yeah, I'm the worst. Good luck.'

That afternoon they were too busy to talk, and as Roz drove away after her shift, leaving Susannah open-mouthed in the car park, she knew her friend wasn't going to let it drop. The parting comment was crystal-clear.

'Tick-tock, Harkin! Tick-tock!' Roz had made a noise like a chicken and laughed like a gurgling drain all the way to her car. Susannah muttered something about friends and enemies under her breath, wondering how she was going to get out of asking Chris on a date without Roz carrying out her threat. She had warmed to Chris now, but dating? No. It just wasn't going to happen. They were far too different. She found him stuffy, and too reserved at times. He thought she was eccentric and gave out such mixed messages that even when she thought she might be feeling something, before she could sound it out in her own head, he was different again—seemingly irritated by her, and showing another side of himself that seemed to come from nowhere. Or he was back in himself again, hidden from her understanding. It had been like Jekyll and Hyde at the beginning, but now she knew more about him, about why he might be like that, it annoyed her that she found him more fascinating as a result.

Two days later, the foster carer called again. Susannah had space now, and the pregnant dog was close to delivery. She needed to be moved now, and Susannah knew just what to do. She would call Chris and have him come to the house. A date of sorts, to keep Roz off her back. Once Susannah had collected the very pregnant and nervous-looking golden retriever—a three-year-old bitch called Melody—she'd already planned the conversation in her head. Once the dog was settled in the utility room, in a large makeshift birthing pen filled with blankets, Susannah left the exhausted and slightly stressed dog to sleep, keeping the door open so she could observe her.

When her friend Trudy came over a couple of hours later, Susannah was on her hands and knees scrubbing the kitchen tiles with a hard-bristled brush. Trudy was another animal foster mum and actual mum of Isabelle, who was fifteen and puppy mad. They looked at the sparkling floor, and back to Susannah.

'You okay? I think it's clean.'

'Oh, hi! Thanks for coming. I don't want to leave her for long but the dogs need a good run outside.' Isabelle was already peering into the utility room, over the safety gate.

'Aww, she's beautiful.'

Trudy smiled at her daughter and peered over the gate at the sleeping dog.

'Aww, yes, she's lovely. Don't you rush;

she'll be fine with us. We've got some school-work to do, haven't we, Issy?' Isabelle groaned. 'Home-schooling, don't you just love it?'

From the look on Trudy's face, Susannah knew it was a bit of an ordeal for them both. Isabelle struggled at school, and, with her autism, the outdoors and animals were the only things that made her really happy, that made her feel like herself. She was going to be following in her mum's footsteps, that was for sure. Trudy had a horse stable, of-fering full livery, and her place was always booked out.

'Well, my computer is in the study, if you want to use the Internet, and I have all kinds of stationery in there. You just help yourself, okay? I made oat muffins too, there on the side.' Isabelle grinned at her, and Susannah winked back. Issy had been a sucker for her oat muffins since she was little.

Trudy walked into the hall, leaving Issy to boot up the computer and log into her on-line lesson.

'What's with all the nervous energy?' she asked as soon as her daughter was out of earshot.

Susannah finished scrubbing the rest of the kitchen floor and snapped off her Marigolds.

'Me? Oh, nothing. I just thought I'd make sure it was ready for Melody, that's all.'

'Uh-huh,' Trudy said non-committally. 'I'm pretty sure *you* could give birth on this floor, never mind Melody. What's eating you?'

'Oh, nothing much. I have to ask a man out, and I don't really want to, but Roz—'

Trudy went to flick on the kettle, getting a can of Coke out of her bag and giving it to her daughter, who was busy rolling her eyes at the teacher on the screen in front of her. She closed the study door a little, and then rounded on her friend.

'Right, we have at least half an hour. The dogs can wait. Spill. What man?'

Trudy had drunk half her tea by the time Susanna had told her all about the vet, the issues hampering her charity-drive rollout, and Roz's threat to out her if she didn't ask Chris out.

'And what's the dirt she's got on you?' Trudy pressed, a wry smile across her features.

'My dancing.'

Trudy tried not to laugh but failed miserably. 'Oh, that Roz, she's a wily one.'

'She's evil incarnate, and she has video evidence.'

Trudy whistled through her teeth.

'Oh, then you're just going to have to do it! It will be fine, I'm sure. You get on, right? You and Chris? I've only met him once. He came to check on Misty. He seemed nice. Misty liked him well enough.'

Misty was her mare, a black horse with white markings that was a bit of a character around the village, known for picking apples off people's trees on her hacks out.

'Well, yeah, now I suppose we do, but there's more to this. He's not in the right place to date anyone.'

Trudy frowned. 'But you are.'

'Yes!' Susannah exclaimed. 'I mean, no! No, well, not on an app anyway. Oh, God, Trude, I don't know.' She sagged down in her chair, hating her own indecision. She wished she could rip it out, like the grey hair she'd yanked out earlier that morning in the mirror. 'Roz has a point, but I'm okay on my own.'

Trudy pointed to the pristine kitchen floor. 'Yeah, sure you are.'

'I was only cleaning!'

Trudy shook her head. 'This isn't cleaning, this is…something else.'

'A bit of obsessive bleaching is hardly a sign of sexual frustration, Trude.'

'No, but it's not as much fun as the alternative, is it? You look great; you're athletic, independent. You have your own house and car. Why wouldn't a man love to meet someone like you? You don't have to go mad with it. A couple of dates won't kill you, Susie.' She eyed the closed study door, where the two women could hear Issy's teacher instructing the class. 'Listen, I would love to have a night out. One where I can dress up and not be Issy's mum. Just for one day. It's not good to be isolated, trust me.'

Susannah felt awful for offloading about her problems to her friend. She knew that Issy's condition meant that Trudy often preferred her own company, and the comforts of home. Trudy was a foster carer because she wanted to keep busy at home. Susannah suddenly felt awful for appearing so selfish.

'I'm sorry, I didn't mean to moan at you.'

Trudy waved her off. 'Don't be daft! I'm happy with my lot, Susie. I have my house, and my work, and Issy is my priority.' She looked around her at the immaculate home that Susannah had cultivated since her divorce. 'You have a lovely life too. I just sometimes wish you would realise that you don't have to be alone if you don't want to be. I'm happily single for now.'

That was the difference, Susannah realised. Trudy was busy with a full life, just like her, but she didn't need anyone else in her life. When Susannah thought of the long winter nights ahead, cosied up indoors with her dogs, she knew that, while it seemed idyllic, it soon lost its appeal. The animals were great, but they didn't talk back. They didn't hold her in their arms after a bad day at work, even as comforting as they were. Hell, even Hendrix had thawed out the vet's heart. If a bit of company could do that for him, surely she could see the merits in trying.

Trudy and Issy went home for lunch once the lessons had finished and Susannah was back from walking the dogs. The long, brisk walk had really helped to clear her head. Trudy and Roz, Helen, Cheryl…they were all so bent on getting her out there. Maybe they had a point. It had been a long time since she'd looked at a male. One without a hairy snout anyway.

She checked on Melody, who was now eating quite happily in her room, and reached for her mobile. The surgery would be closing in half an hour, and she needed to stop talking herself in and out of what she was about to do.

Chris had just waved off the last patient of the day when the mobile in his coat pocket rang. Susannah. He jabbed at the button.

'Don't tell me,' he said with a grin. 'You've rescued a wild cheetah from your back garden, and you want me to clip his nails.'

'Ha ha,' she retorted. 'Very funny.'

The line went quiet, and Chris looked at the display in confusion. 'Susie, you there?'

'Yes, sorry! I'm here. Less of the Susie too. No one calls me that.'

Good, he thought to himself. *I like hearing that. Susie will be sticking, if I have anything to do with it.*

'I think it's rather cute. So, what's up?'

'Nothing.' She sounded weird, and Chris wondered if work had upset her. 'I just wanted to ask you if you would come and check one of the new dogs I have. This one's pregnant, due any day.'

'Well, congratulations! Grandma Harkin, eh?'

Her reply came through gritted teeth. 'Again, very funny. I thought if you were free tonight perhaps I can make a bit of dinner, if you have time.'

'Dinner?' he checked, wondering if his ears were suddenly playing up. 'At your house?'

'Tonight, yes. Only if you have the time, of course.'

Chris looked at the phone display again before answering. He was so shocked he felt the need to check he wasn't being pranked.

'Er, no… I mean, yes, I have the time. That would be great.'

'Really? Oh, that's great, then.'

A lot of greats being thrown around. Awkward.

'Do I need to bring anything?'

'No, just yourself. Maybe your kit bag, for Melody.'

'Melody? Will she be joining us?'

'She's the dog, Chris.'

'Oh! Okay! Just the two of us, then.'

He heard her slight hesitation on the line and pondered for the fifth time that minute what was happening.

'Yes, I guess it is. Just the two of us.' Another long pause. 'Seven, then?'

'Seven's great.'

'Great, see you then?'

'See you then.'

'Bye.'

'Bye.'

'Bye.'

The phone line went dead, but not before he heard the start of what sounded like a groan coming from the other end. A minute later, she rang back.

'Changed your mind?'

'What? Er…no. Why, have you?'

'No, it's been a while since I had a night away from the TV. I do need to come and assess the dog.'

'Of course, yes, I was just ringing back to tell you my address.'

She reeled it off, and he pretended to note it down. The truth was, he'd already looked her up on the computer. Nothing in the realms of stalking, but he had found himself intrigued whenever she'd spoken of her house. Solitary Cottage wasn't a name he was likely to forget.

'Okay, I'll see you tonight, then.'

'Okay, see you soon.' She rang off again, and he was still standing there staring at his phone when Cheryl walked in, coat on and keys in hand.

'Chris, everything okay?'

'Yes.' He smiled. 'Actually, I think I've just been asked on a date.'

Cheryl's face was a picture.

'Really? That's…amazing.'

Chris chuckled, shutting everything down and heading out to Reception with her. Hendrix was already sitting there by the door, his lead in his mouth. He had got to know the drill of working together, and now you could set a clock by the dog.

'Who's the lucky lady?' Cheryl asked as he walked her over to their cars. 'Anyone I know?'

'Melody,' he said with a smile. 'I don't think you've met.'

CHAPTER SIX

HE KNOCKED AT the door and smiled at the cacophony of dogs barking. It was quite remote, he noted, but friendly-looking. The whole place reminded him of her: bright colours everywhere and little homely touches to the gardens and outside of her home that made it easier to walk towards. The place felt like a warm hug, and then the door opened, and she was there.

She looked a little more muted that evening, but that didn't stop her from lighting up the room. He hardly noticed what she was wearing at first. It was her he saw. Her white dress was casual, but fitted her so well it clung to her skin in all the right places. Chris forgot who he was for a second as he took her in. It had a vee neckline, showing off her pale, freckly skin. Her hair was brightened by the white of her dress, and her green eyes stared right at him.

'Hi,' she stammered, hopping from foot to foot. He followed the motion, taking in a pair of shapely legs, long and beautiful. Her slender ankles were encased in…in…

'Hi. I like your slippers.' Her face dropped, and she looked down in dismay at her novelty unicorn slippers. 'Cute.' She had flushed, and it made her eyes all the more noticeable. He had to keep looking away to keep his balance.

She doesn't always look like this. What's the deal?

'Yeah, present from a workmate. I forgot to change. Come on in.' She noticed the wine in his hands, and the kit bag. 'Oh, is that for us?'

'Well, the kit bag's for the dog, and this is to say thanks for the meal.'

'You haven't eaten it yet.' She beamed, taking the wine and kicking the slippers off her feet into the corner. 'Do you want to sit first, or see Melody?'

He knew she already knew what he'd say. 'Lead the way.' He lifted his medical bag.

The utility room was nice and warm, and the bedding she'd kitted out was pretty plush. He sat next to the pen for a moment, letting Melody make her way over and sniff him out. Animals didn't like feeling cornered; they were much like humans in that respect. He could already tell from a visual inspection that she was due any time, and looked healthy and well, if a little underweight. She'd already been bathed and treated for fleas. Her bites were healing nicely, the fur starting to grow back well. He'd need to carry out all the checks to make sure the delivery would be a smooth one. A thought occurred to him.

'Do you have a birthing partner in mind?'

If Susannah was startled by the question, she didn't show it. 'Well, it depends on the shifts I'm on. Most of my cover options have people at home they care for, and others work shifts too. We make it work, but I might be a little bit stuck on this one.

'When are you working next?'

'Tomorrow. First of four night shifts. We've had a few people promoted or gone to other jobs. HR messed up, so we're all pulling in extras when we can. Melody was checked over but the pups weren't spotted so this is all a bit of a last-minute situation.'

Chris rolled his eyes. 'What vet missed that?'

Susannah shrugged. 'I don't know. Not as easy as peeing on a stick, I suppose. Some of the dogs are so traumatised when they come in, and…' She trailed off with a smile. 'Of course, you know. I'll let you get on; she seems to have accepted you.' Melody was now licking Chris's hand, much to Susannah's surprise and delight. He did have a way with the animals. It made her think of what her mother used to tell her. Her father had always been a huge dog lover, and it had always given her mum such joy to see them together. She'd always said that animals were a great judge of character, and Chris, even with his moods, had charmed every animal she'd seen him with. He definitely didn't tally with the first opinions of the villagers of his bedside manner.

When he'd finished, he headed into the kitchen, where Susannah was at the stove.

'Do you think she'll last till after my shifts?'

'I don't think so. It'll be any time now really. Have you not got a foster that could take her?'

'No, I took her as an emergency case as it is. I can make it work. You ready to eat? It's just my beef stew, but I have been told it's quite tasty.'

The table in the kitchen was laid out simply, not romantic as such, but it was certainly cosy. She placed a stew pot at the centre of the table on a warmer, putting down hunks of buttered crusty bread. The wine was on the side in an ice bucket, and as he entered the room and washed up she lit a couple of candles around the room. He felt his eyebrows rise. Candles? With him? Maybe this was something. A real date? No, couldn't be. Could it?

'It smells amazing, thanks. I'll get the wine.' He'd already noted the empty wine glasses on the table. His stomach was gurgling, and the smell of her home, coupled with the tempting food, made him feel rather comforted. It was a while since he'd spent an evening like this.

'How's Hendrix?' she asked as she sat down next to him at the table. He was pouring the wine, and he gave her a cheeky grin.

'I left him with the remote. Told him not to try to watch any pay-per-view.'

'Ha ha,' she retorted. 'Will he be okay on his own?'

'He'll be fine. I would have brought him but I figured you have enough on.' He held his wine glass aloft as she started to spoon the stew onto their plates. 'God, that looks amazing. Shall we have a toast?'

Susannah, already confused by his rather chipper mood, looked at him quizzically, her own glass raised now.

'If you like. What are we drinking to?'

'Oh, I don't know. Good food, good company. We have the village hall meeting on Monday evening.'

'So you want to say cheers to an event that I basically forced you to take part in?' she said drily. Chris looked at her amused face and blushed.

'Well, yes. I say we cheers to the charity drive, and to the dogs.' He pinned her with his gaze over his glass. 'I know we didn't have the best start, but I do see how valued your work is. The kennel work, I mean.' He cleared his throat, pushing his glass closer to hers in the air. She didn't touch her glass to his, holding it away instead.

'Well, I would say that all the work I do is valued.'

His eyes didn't leave hers when he answered.

'I didn't say it wasn't.'

'Well, it was implied. I know you have an issue with my being a nurse, but—'

'I don't have an issue with you being a nurse. When did I say that? I don't pick on other professions.'

'I know, but with your wife and everything.'

'Karen? What does she have to do with this?' His nostrils flared, and Susannah lowered her glass.

She felt like necking the whole thing down. It had started so well. She'd cleaned the house, put on a nice outfit. She had reasoned with herself that while she had been a bit shifty about this 'date' with Chris, she could use the opportunity to see how dating would feel. Judging by the fact that they'd not even lifted a fork, and were already quarrelling, she knew the evening would be a bit less fun than she'd thought. Mr Hyde was here again, it seemed, and he was ripping a slice of bread into smaller and smaller pieces with his fingers. As if it were a murder victim he were disembowelling. He noticed her watching, and huffily he stilled his hands. She took a sip of her wine and picked up her cutlery.

She'd only just taken a mouthful when he spoke again.

'I'm sorry. I didn't mean to make things awkward.'

'I know.'

'I just don't like talking about any of it.'

'I know that too.' She lowered her fork. 'The thing is, sometimes you have to.'

His jaw clenched, but she pressed on.

'Tell me something about Karen—nothing medical or sad. You must have good times you remember.'

He sat back in his chair, running his hand through his hair. It left it tufted up at odd angles, softening his look now he'd seemingly lost his flash of anger. Susannah watched as he composed himself, practically seeing the grief winding around his body like a wisp of smoke. He needed to talk about it, realise his anger.

'She wouldn't have liked it here, in Puddle Lake.'

Susannah smiled, sitting back and eating some of her stew. She wanted him to talk and not feel gawked at. 'Really. City girl, eh?'

Chris smiled. 'Oh, yeah. She would never consider something like this to be interesting enough. She needed top Wi-Fi, good coffee shops, and access to work. We were both like that really, but I always thought about slowing down.'

'What did she do?'

'She was a solicitor. We met at university. We ended up with a bunch of mutual friends, and we all just kind of went through it together. A few of us paired off.'

'Driven woman; I'm impressed. Sounds like you had a lot of fun.'

'We did.' He seemed to be remembering that himself. 'We did, yeah.'

'Good. Eat your stew; it'll get cold.'

They sat and ate in silence for a while, the dogs all seemingly asleep now. Chris checked in on Melody, and Susannah refilled her wine while he was gone. She held out the bottle in his direction when he retook his seat. He took it from her and filled his glass.

'Thanks. She's fast asleep. I think we're safe for tonight.'

Susannah puffed out a breath, blowing strands of hair across her face. She blew again to dispel them and saw that he was smiling at her.

'What?'

'You make me laugh.'

Susannah's brows were up in her hairline, and that made him laugh again. 'You do! It's true. I'm used to you now.'

'You make me sound like an old sock or something,' she countered with a huff.

'You're very expressive.' He pointed his finger in a circle in front of her face. 'Like Jim Carrey.'

'Jim Carrey is a man.'

'I'm well aware of that. I only mean his rather rubbery face. You look like that.' The finger ran in circles again. She pretended to snap at it with her teeth, and he jumped back, sloshing his own wine over his shirt. He cursed loudly, grabbing one of the tea towels hung up nearby and dabbing at his chest. Susannah watched the whole thing and tried not to giggle.

'Sorry,' she tried to get out, but the end of the word dissolved into laughter. 'Oh, God, sorry! I always laugh at things like that. Nervous response. Take your shirt off.'

'What?' Chris was trying to rub the stain into submission.

'Your shirt will stain, you're all wet, and you stink of booze. Take it off, put your jacket back on. I can bob it in the washer.' She looked towards the utility room where a sleeping Melody could be seen. She nibbled her lip. Too noisy. 'Or I can hand wash it?'

Chris had no shirt on when she turned back to him, and for a second she couldn't breathe. The shock of his naked chest, in her kitchen, with the candles and the 'date' vibes, hit her all at once. He was ripped underneath his shirt. She'd kind of had an idea that he was well toned. He walked a certain way, with a confident stride. She had once thought it was a swagger, but she knew now he was just built that way. And he had the goods to back it up.

'I'll just take it home.' He grinned, and then he covered himself up with his jacket, leaving it unbuttoned. When she sat back down across from him she could still see a bit of his rather sculpted torso. It was very distracting. 'Thanks though. I didn't mean the Jim Carrey thing as an insult.'

'Oh?' Susannah forced her eyes back up to his chest. 'I don't have a rubber face, then?' She'd forgotten about his awkward observation. She was still lusting after his body. There was so much more to this guy than she'd first thought.

I'm actually enjoying myself.

'Yes. No. Wow, I am always tongue-tied around you.'

She snorted when she laughed this time. 'What? As if!'

'I am—you're too quick sometimes.'

'Well, you mumble.'

'I don't think I do.'

'Sorry, was that doo-doo-tink-a-do?' She held her hand over her mouth, speaking through it and muffling her voice. He laughed, giving her a playful shove with his hand.

'Sarcasm is the lowest form of wit, you know.'

'Yeah, but it's worth it for the laugh. You're not tongue-tied around me; I could say the same though. You were rough when I first met Hendrix.'

'Rough? I don't think I was that bad. Not oafish, anyway.'

Susannah's eyes narrowed. 'Oafish?'

He waved his hand, reaching for another slice of bread to mop up the remnants of the gravy. 'Oh, yeah, apparently one of my clients called me an oaf.' He clicked his fingers. 'A bullish oaf, that was it.'

She cleared her throat. 'Well, I bet whoever it was thought their feedback would have been kept confidential. Cheryl has a big mouth.' She huffed under her breath, and Chris's eyes snapped to hers.

'It was you!'

'Yes!' she admitted, covering her face with one of her hands and transferring gravy onto her cheek. She rubbed it off with a napkin. 'I did. I'm sorry. You were a bit of an oaf though.'

He opened his mouth to argue but smiled instead. 'Okay, yes. I'll give you that one.' He continued to mop up the last of the gravy. Susannah rose to her feet, reaching into the fridge for dessert.

'Thanks. I will kill Cheryl when I see her next.'

'Oh, no, don't do that. I couldn't run the

practice without her. Why don't I help with Melody?'

He was collecting the dishes from the table now, and he opened the dishwasher to start stacking the empty plates.

'You? I can do that.' He shrugged and kept going. 'You can't help really; it's nights I need the help for.'

'Don't be daft. It's the least I can do. Goodness, that looks nice.' She was cutting slices of the Oreo cheesecake she'd made for the evening. 'Did you make that?'

'Yep. It's full of sugar but it tastes like heaven.' She grabbed a fork, spearing a corner of one slice and holding it up for him to try. He came closer, and she could smell the spicy scent of his aftershave. It suited him. Woodsy, strong. He leaned in, taking the morsel of cake from her fork. She found herself watching his lips, and he groaned in pleasure.

'Wow. I can feel my arteries hardening already, but what a way to go.' He waggled his eyebrows at her, and she giggled, taking a bite herself.

'Mmm, that is good.' They took it over to the table, not bothering with plates. Chris took another big scoop on his fork and tucked in. 'I wish I'd made two now. The girls at work would love this.'

'Do you often bake for the hospice?'

She raised a brow at his mention of the hospice, but she answered quickly.

'Yeah, I get bored some evenings.' She looked around her home, which was neat and bright, just like her. 'I love the cottage, but it's not exactly on a busy street. Once I'm in for the night with the dogs, the time can be a bit hard to fill.'

'I know what you mean. I have my work, of course, and Hendrix now. He's a little turd, but it has made me realise how introverted I've become. Walking him round here, I've met more people than I did in the city.'

'Well, that's Puddle Lake for you. We all live in each other's pockets, but we're nice to each other. It works. What do you do when you're not working?'

His blank face said it all. 'Not much, to be honest. Which is why I can help with Melody. I can watch her while you're on nights.'

'I can't move her though. It would be too distressing for her to move again.'

'I know, but I can come here. If you don't mind me sleeping on your couch of course.'

A man on my couch. That sounds so alien.

'I have a spare room, but I couldn't ask you to do that. What about Hendrix?'

'I can bring him with me. I'm sure he won't be any trouble. It means I'll be here if the pups come in the night. You can concentrate on your work.'

'I can't ask you to do that.'

He put his hand over hers. 'You didn't ask, and you did feed me tonight. Throw in another cheesecake when you're baking next, and we'll call it quits. Cheryl and the girls will love me if I bring one of these in.' He waggled his loaded fork at her, but she was looking at their joined hands. Chris coughed and pulled his away to reach for the wine bottle. 'We're nearly out. Just as well—I have the car.' He hiccupped. 'I might get a taxi anyway, actually. Mind if I leave the car?'

Since she'd already done the same to him, she nodded. 'No problem. Are you really sure about Melody though?'

'Of course. She's my patient. It will cost you to keep her in the practice overnight, and I have nothing on. As long as you don't mind me being in your house alone.'

She had a sudden image of him taking in her rather eclectic decorating, but she did need the help. The thought of having a vet in her house, looking after the dogs and Melody, flooded her with a great sense of relief.

'I'm okay with that, but I couldn't ask it of you.'

'You didn't ask, remember? I'll come after work tomorrow night and you can show me what's what.' He'd demolished two large pieces of cheesecake, and he patted his non-existent stomach with a frown. 'I'll have to walk that lot off. I'm stuffed. Thank you.'

'You're welcome. It's the least I owe you, what with the charity drive.'

'I know, we haven't even talked about that. Don't you think we should get our ducks in a row before the meeting?'

Susannah groaned. 'I have a huge file—it's in the sitting room.' She looked at the time; it was still quite early. 'Do you need to get off? We can go through it now, if you like.' He was still patting his stomach and stifling a belch. She tried and failed not to laugh. 'I have more wine, and some Pepto if you need it. I am grateful, you know, for all your help. I know I'm stubborn.'

'Me too. I know I wasn't my best when we first met. I was a bit mad.' He tilted his head to the lounge. 'Shall we get some planning done, then?' Rising to his feet, he took the glass from her hand with his.

Her lounge was as neat as always. A book lay across the arm of her reading chair, the blanket lying haphazardly across it. She had two lamps lighting the room, and the fire was lit. It looked rather cosy, and she caught his expression as he took in the room. She took a seat on the large couch, the oversized cushions all bearing funny slogans.

'It's very you, this room.' He seduced her with a slow-burning smile before sitting down next to her. She spread the file out on the coffee table in front of them. 'Wow. So is that file.'

She rolled her eyes at him. 'Yeah yeah, I'm slightly bonkers and highly organised. I've been told. Do you want to do this or not?' She jostled him with her elbow, laughing when he pretended to be mortally wounded. 'Stop being a jerk.'

'A jerk now, eh? That's an improvement from oaf.'

She nudged him again, and he nudged her back this time. They were nose to nose now, and she was laughing her head off. It was a minute before she realised he'd stopped laughing. He'd also moved closer.

'This might be the wine talking, but I love to hear you laugh.' He looked at her in a way he never had before. 'You irritate the hell out of me—' he ignored her pout '—but you brighten my day, Susannah. Your laugh, it's something I always look forward to.'

She didn't quite know what to say, but he did.

'I've really enjoyed our date. I wanted to say that before we start talking about Portaloos.'

She burst into guffaws of laughter. He watched her with a very amused smile on his face. His hair was a little messed up, making him look more casual than usual. Ruffled.

'You're a goofball deep down, do you know that?'

'Yep. Just like you.' He looked her up and down slowly. 'Minus the colourful clothing.' He bit at his lip. 'I'm not all bad. I wish you'd known me before, when I was younger. I was different then.'

'Things change us in life,' she soothed.

'Nothing's changed you.'

She laughed again. 'Not now, no. It took me a while after my divorce to lick my wounds. I bought this place and just hid away at first.'

'Doesn't sound like you.'

He spoke as if he'd known her much longer than he had, but it sounded right to her too. They had seemingly been studying each other. Judged each other, yelled at each other, but yet here they were laughing, working on the charity drive together and enjoying the evening.

'It wasn't,' she breathed. 'I'm glad you came to live here. I'm not sure if anyone's actually said that to you yet.'

'It is nice to hear.' He was so close now. His eyes were taking her in, and she felt the stirrings of attraction sparking. 'Especially from you.'

'Your harshest critic,' she near whispered. They laughed again. 'What a battle-scarred pair we are.'

He laughed softly again, and something changed. It was so slight, so minuscule that she could easily have missed it, but he tore his gaze from hers, and poured them both a glass of wine.

'We'd better get on with the planning, then—I need to get back to Hendrix.' He wasn't rude, or surly. He was the man she'd come to know. The man who was so but-toned-up, she didn't think he'd ever get free. She hid her red face behind her wine glass, taking a good long pull. Trudy was coming to sort the dogs tomorrow, so she could sleep all day and then hide in work. Then she hid her disappointment at the date that wasn't a date. The non-date that had turned into a hot date and then back into a non-date. Just as she was starting to feel…

Well, it wasn't anything, obviously. She sat up on her couch, pulled a pen from the pile on the table, and flipped open her notepad. Closing her heart at the same time.

'It was just a planning meeting and a meal, Roz.'

'It went well. Must be off, busy day!'

'Roz, mind your own beeswax, you nosy co—'

Maybe not. Susannah huffed into the mirror. The staffroom was compact but neat and she was alone. She was very early for the start of her shift, driven out by Chris arriving to look after Melody. She'd been writing and deleting texts cancelling him all day, but she had to admit that it was pretty stupid to turn down a free overnight vet on call. She had to put Melody first, and what would she say as an excuse anyway? The rest of the night had been cordial enough—they'd even laughed— but there was an awkward distance between them now. Him hiding his obvious pain and her smarting from the rejection. She didn't even think he knew it was a rejection, and that was the worst part. He'd had a moment with her—she'd been able to tell when he'd looked at her that he'd felt something like she had—but they had both taken very different paths with the information.

And so, she'd been ready when he'd arrived at her house, bag in hand, instructions on the counter with her work number and other information. She'd gone overboard, but when she'd woken up that late afternoon, she'd been possessed with a need to get organised—her old trick for helping cheer herself up, and to feel in control. She knew her own behaviours well enough now, but it had given her the resolve to be normal around him. She'd been nice and friendly, laughing and joking, thanking him. She'd even cooked for him, labelling everything up in the fridge. She'd set out a basket for Hendrix too, so he'd feel at home at the cottage. She couldn't be mad at a man who didn't even know he'd upset her, let alone an innocent dog caught in the crossfire.

She'd always known he was grieving. She didn't have an excuse for feeling a bit sorry for herself. She'd gone against her golden rule of never being second best again, but he was someone she liked being around. He'd told her the same that night. They had the dogs and the charity drive together; it was too complicated to just ignore the man for the rest of her life. She'd have to move out of the village, and she wasn't about to over-react like that. Not yet, anyway.

She'd felt the same flicker of attraction as she'd left her house. He'd leaned in to kiss her cheek, wishing her a happy shift and telling her to be careful driving. It had felt so nice to see him again, and he had looked good. So she'd fled to work, smiling and waving like an idiot as he'd stood there outside her house, waving her off with her dogs and Hendrix milling around his feet. She'd driven away so fast she'd nearly chipped her windscreen on the shale. Once she was out of sight, she'd cursed herself for being such a goof over the complicated man again. Now she was here at work, and she knew that Roz would try to interrogate her after handover. She straightened her curls into a bright green hair tie, and made herself a cup of tea before the other night staff arrived.

As it went, handover was quite busy. They'd had a lot to report, and Roz had been so tired she'd just hugged her and left to get home to her bed. The night shift was busy too, with lots of monitoring and care needed, and she'd not even thought about anything else other than the job since her shift started. She took her break in the staffroom, wishing she could have the coffee in her hand administered by drip. She retrieved her phone from her locker, checking her messages. Friends, a few junk emails for dating sites and dog-food offers. Damn the intelligent advertising these days; you looked up something once, and that was all they tried to sell you for the next six months. It was depressing. She noticed a message from him.

Melody is comfortable, but I can tell she's getting a bit moody. I think she'll deliver tomorrow night. How much do you bet? Dogs all fine. Thanks for the food. That pasta thing was amazing. Hope work is going well.

It was nice to think of him texting her from her little house, keeping the dogs company. She rested her tea next to her snack on the table next to her, and tapped out a reply.

Thanks for looking after them. I know better than to bet against a vet on matters like this. You're welcome. Chilli tomorrow night?

Sour cream?

Sure. Sorry if I woke you. She'd belatedly realised the time of night, or early morning, it
was.

You didn't. I'll bring dessert.

Deal.

That was all she wrote back, after deleting her rather saucier reply. It was easy to fall
into that easy to and fro with him, though.
It was nice.

A deal or a bet?

Oh. So he was teasing now.

Deal for the pudding, no bet on Melody. I
think you're right.

She'd seen enough pregnant and labour-
ing dogs in her time to recognise the signs.

Can I get that in writing, please?

You just did. That's all I can do. How come
you're still up?

Woke up. The spare room is choking me with its sunshine décor.

She laughed. It was a little bright, but it was a guest room. Obviously she wanted it to cheer her guests up. She giggled at the thought of him in it. Mr grey suit. She tapped back, checking the clock.

I need to get back. Don't moan about my taste, your house could use a splash of colour. Ha ha.

He replied straight away, and she felt the thrill hit her when her phone pinged again.

You shall have to teach me. We could go shopping? Lunch in it for you.

What? Was this a date? After last time… She only had a couple of minutes left. She rammed everything she had left into her mouth, trying to think of a quick reply. One that would find out the situation without *asking* about the situation.

She was still chewing when her phone beeped again. She jumped, scrabbling to read the message.

It doesn't have to be a date.

That was it. So he had picked up on the change in the air the other night. She knew it know. He was giving her an out. And now she was due back, and she still hadn't replied. She didn't open the text on her phone this time, so he couldn't tell that she'd read it. She'd pretend she was back on shift instead. It would give her time to think of an answer. Turning her phone off, she tried to push it out of her mind. Back to work.

No reply.

Chris woke up in Susannah's spare room and the first thing he did was check his phone. She'd not replied to his last two texts, and he had a feeling that whatever this was, he'd just messed it up. He wasted no time in getting ready for work, making sure he left everything clean and in order. He went and saw to all the dogs, checking in on Melody, who tucked into her breakfast with encouraging gusto. Hendrix was as loopy as ever, running around in the yard with the other dogs like an utter nutcase. He sat on one of the chairs on the patio area to drink his coffee and watch them, waiting for Susannah to walk in to relieve him. He'd used her coffee machine, long neglected in the corner, and had a bubbling pot of the fresh good stuff waiting for her. He knew she liked her caffeine. He'd even put the teapot on standby in case she wanted that.

He was feeling good about helping her, and the realisation that he did care had loosened something in him. They were friends, so why not date? She was so nice; they got on. He knew without a shadow of a doubt that he was attracted to her. Being so close the other night had spooked him, but only because of the depth of his feelings. He'd wanted to take her into his arms and kiss the hell out of her, but he'd screwed it up. It was becoming a pattern: she'd get close, he'd gnash his teeth and snap at her ankles. He was like a battle-scarred rescue dog. Maybe that was what she saw in him. It wasn't a good look to have, especially given the fact that he did want to kiss her. In fact, it was pretty much all he thought about. Which then brought on the guilt spasms in his chest, and made him think of Karen, and then he was angry and glum all over again. And so the cycle continued.

He checked his phone. Still nothing. He sat watching the dogs till he saw her car come up the long driveway, and then he girded his loins and went to meet her.

'Hi.' She yawned in his face. 'Ooh, sorry.'

'You look really tired. Bad shift?'

'Not bad so much as busy. We had a lot on and the call buttons were pretty continuous. I hope the day shift got some sleep. It was still a bit manic when I left.' She walked into the kitchen, spotting the coffee and half running to it. 'Oh, my God, I love you!' She whirled around, a fresh mug still in hand, her face a picture of embarrassment. 'You know what I mean. I didn't even know how to work this thing. This is amazing!' She was lifting the coffee pot on and off the hot plate in wonder. Filling her cup, she sipped at it with both hands wrapped around the mug. 'Dear Lord, that's the stuff.'

'You really like your coffee.' His lips pulled into a smirk.

'The darker the better.' She nodded her head at her mug. 'This should just about give me the energy to climb the stairs. How's Melody?'

'Still pregnant, and a bit flatulent as well. She ponged out your utility room.'

Susannah smiled, stifling another yawn.

'I'll let you get to bed. I'll see you tonight.' He bent in and touched his lips to hers. It was so quick she didn't get time to respond. 'Sleep well.'

He threw her a sexy final look and then, calling to Hendrix, he got into his car and headed off down the drive. She watched until he lost sight of her. It had been impulsive, the peck, but he hadn't been able to help himself. He'd needed to do it, and he hadn't regretted it. Before he got home, his phone beeped. He read the text from its cradle on the dashboard as he neared home wearily.

Yes, it's a date.

She'd texted back. The second he was parked on his drive, he grabbed his phone and typed one back, grinning like an idiot.

Glad to hear. it. You looked beautiful this morning. See you tonight.

CHAPTER SEVEN

'MRS CHAN AND little Gustav! How lovely to see you today!'

Mrs Chan set the cat carrier on the floor and picked up her chin. She gawped at Chris as he smiled back at her.

'What's wrong with you?'

'Me?' Chris gestured to himself with his thumbs. 'Nothing, why?'

'You're so…cheerful. It's weird.' She flipped open the cage door, and hoisted Gustav onto the table. Chris took in the cat's new slightly thinner frame and his smile grew.

'Well, I'm just so happy that Gustav here is finally on the way to being able to reach his little kitty bits. Well done, Mrs Chan—he looks great.'

'Are you being sarcastic? It's been really hard—he gives me these big sad eyes—but I stuck to it. I gave all his treats to the shelter; he didn't speak for me for two days.'

'No sarcasm here—it's the lowest form of wit. You are looking after him really well, Mrs Chan. I mean that. It's only been a few weeks, but I can already see the difference. He's going to be one happy cat come bikini-wearing time.'

She was looking at him quizzically one minute, and then he was being cuddled over the table.

'Thanks, Doctor. I thought you were a bit of a git when you first came, but you're not all bad.'

'Thanks, Mrs Chan. Tell your friends, eh, ask them to lower their pitchforks?'

'Ha!' she exploded. 'That's pretty funny. I will see what I can do.'

She was still chuckling when he'd finished the examination. His day went like a breeze. All of his clients and their owners were happy. He was the best veterinarian he'd ever been, and he hoped this feeling would last. It was Susannah, he realised. She'd quite literally come bounding into his life and sprayed it with colour. He was looking forward to seeing her that night, before she left for work. He liked staying in her house too—not that he was snooping or anything untoward. He just felt peaceful there, with her stuff all around. She made him food and left it for him. He felt cared for, and it was rather nice.

Karen had been fiercely independent in that way too, but she'd never showed her care for him that way. Both driven by their work, but expressing it in different ways. But unlike Karen, Susannah found joy in other things— in people and animals. She seemed to want to help the whole world, and he wondered who showed her care. He knew her friends and the community loved her because there were photos of them all around and little notes on the fridge from them. She was obviously loved, but alone. As he was. It was just them and their dogs, and now each other. He didn't know how to process the feelings he was having, but he wanted to go with them. She was changing him, changing his world, and it felt good.

As he locked up that evening, seeing his colleagues to their cars and heading off to his with Hendrix, he found his brain picking at his happiness. He had compared her to Karen. He knew he'd done it before too, which was only natural since he was now effectively dating Susannah. The problem was, he was comparing them, when they were total opposites. It wasn't that he was finding one woman better than the other; that was not even in the equation. He'd loved Karen dearly, and they had been wrapped in their own happy little life, busy, ever moving, ever achieving, but then she'd got sick, and when she passed, he'd known that that life was done. It was another life entirely, compared to the one he led now.

Karen had never been one for pets, with their work schedules, and now he had the loopy Hendrix at home. He was living in a picture-postcard village. He'd changed, he realised. His wants and needs had sharpened and were now focused on a quiet life, and work. Then Susannah had come along, and they'd skirted around each other, and now he was dating her, and sleeping in her house to be on puppy watch. Was it the affection she showed to everyone that he craved? Was she a rebound? He didn't know, but he knew his feelings for her were growing stronger. He needed to work it out before he hurt her, or even himself. It hadn't exactly been plain sailing to get to this point. The irony was that he and Karen had talked about work too much, and he and Susannah didn't talk about it at all. There was a part of her life that he didn't want to know about so much. It was a barrier he didn't know how to cross. He gunned the engine for home, eager to get changed, and get to Susannah's. He knew that looking at her would sort his feelings out. He was different around her, but he was still himself. He just needed to be woken up. She'd certainly done that.

'Hendrix, I think we have a lot of work to do.'

Hendrix barked in the back, and it felt like approval.

'Hello? Susie?'

'In the utility room! Oh, thank God you're here. Can you keep Hendrix away?'

Chris dropped the shopping bag, grabbing his kit and shooing Hendrix outside to play in the back garden. Running to the utility room, he saw Susannah in a very short night-robe, and a pair of silky white slippers. Her hair was pinned back haphazardly, and she looked stressed.

'Everything okay?' He dropped to his knees by her side, snapping on a pair of gloves and sanitising both his hands and hers. He noticed she was shaking.

'I couldn't leave her to get my phone. There's too much blood, isn't there?'

Chris shushed her. 'It's a little more than I'd like, but don't panic. You go and get changed, and I'll assess her.' She didn't take her eyes off Melody, and he could see the worry on her face. 'Susie,' he said again. His eyes finally caught hers. 'I've got her. You get ready for work.'

Once she was out of sight, he got to work. The minute he examined Melody, he knew she had a problem.

'Oh, Melody, you poor girl. Let's get your baby out, eh? He's got himself a little bit stuck.' The bleeding was from the straining around the pup. He got to work, being as gentle as possible and checking for any more blood loss. When the pup was out, he put it in front of the mother for her to work her magic. She was panting far less now, and started licking the new arrival. The puppy was out of its sac and cleaned up by the time the next one came. Susannah walked in, looking put together but terrified.

'She's okay. Two so far—Melody's a champ.'

'Really? Thank God for that. She was making some awful noises; I didn't want to touch her and make it worse.'

'You did the right thing. The bleeding was caused when the first little pup got stuck.' He pointed out the bigger of the two healthy-looking puppies. 'I've called him Tank. He's a bit of a beast.'

Susannah grabbed Chris and dropped a very grateful kiss on his lips.

'Thank you. I was worried.'

'Thank you. That was nice. Do I get one for each pup?'

She smiled, rolling her eyes. She leaned in all the same, and when her lips touched his, he pulled her into his arms a bit closer. This kiss was a little longer.

Melody was feeding her pups when they looked in on them. Tank really was living up to his name, guzzling away with his siblings.

'You do know your top's on inside out, don't you?'

She looked down and groaned.

'Oh, God, that would have been bad. Turning up to work like that. Roz would have had a field day. Do you want a coffee, before I go?'

Chris closed the door to the utility room a little but stayed close by to monitor them.

'Please. I brought some bits; I'll just nip and get them from the car while you're here.' He was almost at the front door when he turned back.

'Why would Roz have a field day about a wonky top?'

'Eh?' She was studying the kettle now as if wishing for a genie. 'Oh, you know.'

She could tell from his words that he was smiling.

'No, you'll have to fill me in.'

She sighed dramatically. 'I thought you might. She knows you're helping with Melody, that's all.'

'Ah, and of course, any vet call ends in a wonky-top situation.' His voice was closer now.

'No, I didn't mean that.'

'What did you mean?'

He was teasing her now, and his voice was closer still. She was pretending to be a barista-level coffee-maker to avoid looking him in the eye but he was beside her, and the jig was up.

'Do your friends know about me, then?' He was grinning like a schoolboy, and she didn't know whether to kiss or slap the smirk out of him. 'Me, you and possible wonky-top scenarios?'

She giggled, trying to push her lips together to stop the laughter. They were both so close now, the coffee forgotten. Almost nose to nose.

'Well, we haven't talked about that.' Much.

'But you do talk about me?'

'Well, yes, we are dating. Right?' Her confidence seemed to wane with the end of the sentence.

'Right. I do think we need to talk a little more about what that means at some point.'

'I agree.'

'Definitely more talking about wonky tops too,' he murmured. 'I'll nip to the car.' His eyes flashed as he leaned in to kiss her. She drew him in for a longer caress. Having his mouth on hers thrilled her every time, and she deepened the kiss, testing her feelings. And his, if she was honest. He responded to her fire with fire. They were both snogging, hard, against the kitchen counter. His arms were everywhere, her hands were on his, and only the ringing of her mobile stopped them…after a minute of trying rather steadfastly to ignore it.

'It might be work.' She groaned, pulling away reluctantly. She answered, panting, and he was looking at her, so full of ardour and surprise, the same emotions she was feeling. It made her want to throw her phone over her shoulder and run at him like a sexually starved vixen. Wonky top going the same way as her phone, over her shoulder.

'Hello? Roz?'

'Hi, love, any pups yet?'

'Wha—? Er…yeah…' Chris looked at her ruefully and headed past her to check on Melody.

'Roz!' she whisper-shouted, with that great talent women had. 'What's up?'

'Nothing! Why are you panting?'

'I was er…busy.'

'Busy or *busy*, busy?' She positively leered over the last two words.

'Busy with new puppies.'

'Hmm-hmm. Okay, well, I was just checking in.'

'Checking up, more like.'

'That too. See you soon!'

'Bye. You suck, by the way.'

'Ah, come on. You needed a nudge, yes?'

She heard Chris come back into the room, pulling the shopping out of the bag he'd brought.

'Yes,' she said begrudgingly into the phone. 'I did. I'll be there for handover.'

They ate a quick early supper together. He'd brought some bread and cheeses, thick local ham, olives and local pressed juice to wash it down with. Everything she loved to eat. When she left for work, he kissed her softly at the door, and waved her off. She couldn't even remember driving to work, but when she got there, she couldn't stop smiling. Roz was thrilled, and she didn't even try to rib her friend. Roz was too busy congratulating her on how good and happy she looked.

She did feel great. He was so different from who she'd thought he was. The passion earlier... Well, she had no qualms in that area. Not any more. She fancied him rotten, and she knew the feeling was mutual. When she went on break, he'd already texted her some photos. The puppies had now increased to seven, Tank still being the easily recognisable one out of the bunch with his bulk and the shape of his rather meaty head. Melody was looking good, and Chris had reported that she'd done really well. She messaged him back as she ate a fruit salad as fast as she could. She was still a little full from the supper he'd brought.

So cute. Thank you so much, Chris. I really appreciate it. Will buy you lunch when we go shopping.

As ever, he was quick to text back.

Sounds like a plan. Does that mean my bill won't get paid? I have a hungry dog to feed now you know. Do these little ones have homes lined up?

Susannah laughed, but it didn't last when she thought of the seven new homes she'd have to find. The charity-drive meeting couldn't come soon enough.

Nope, Melody has but the pups will have to be the star attraction of the drive. Another load of homes for us to sweet-talk our way into.

We can do it. Have a good shift, I need to get some shut-eye. Drive home safe.

I will.

She knew it was a slip of the thumb, him calling her home 'home' like that, but it gave her a warm, cosy feeling all the same. She'd forgotten what it was like to share her space with someone. He'd only been there two nights, but it was making her think that this dating thing wouldn't be that bad after all. In fact, if she didn't overthink it, she was actually pretty stoked. Enter Helen.

They'd been working together on a patient, a quiet little gentleman called Freddie, who needed regular through-the-night turns and care. They chatted to him as they worked, telling him what they were doing at every step.

'You have a pressure sore here still, Freddie.' Susannah softly tapped her finger twice on his left hip, and he turned slowly to look where she was pointing. Fred was a man of very few words—near silent, in fact. He used to be a jazz musician before he got ill, playing in venues around the world. Now he spent hours listening to the radio, playing songs on his iPad and filling the room with guitars and strings. He nodded once, wincing as the two women removed the dressing, cleaned out the wound and applied barrier cream to make him more comfortable. 'It's healing well; another week or so and you'll be back on your feet.' Early onset Alzheimer's had caused him to have a fall at home, resulting in a hip fracture and a lengthy stay in hospital. He was mending well, and Susannah could see his colour was looking better. It gave her hope that he would be on his feet again, if only for a little while with his fast-failing health.

Freddie nodded away at her with a distant smile on his face, his ears filled with the sound of his songs. Once he was settled in a comfortable position, and they were cleaning everything away, the chatter turned to all things men.

'So, Roz said you deleted the app, but you still look like the cat that got the cream,' Helen said.

Susannah pulled Freddie's door to a little, heading to the medication cart to ready for the next patient. As she double-checked her list as always, she tried to studiously ignore the question.

'Earth to Nurse Harkin!'

She lifted her eyes over the clipboard. 'I heard you, and now I'm ignoring you.'

'Oh, come on! I know something's going on. Roz has been cagey all week and you look like you've been inhaling fairy dust. Who's the guy?'

Susannah rolled her eyes, but gave in.

'Okay,' she said, finishing her task and heading to the office with Helen at her side. 'It's Chris, the vet. We're dating.' Helen's eyes were like saucers when she sneaked a peek. 'It's new; I don't really want to talk about it. You know Puddle Lake. It's not the greatest place to keep a secret. It's complicated, okay?' She rambled on about privacy, and the village gossip mill. All the while Helen was looking as if she was holding herself together. Rather unsuccessfully too. She looked half mad.

'Do you need to pee or something?'

'No!' Helen jigged from one foot to the other. 'I'm just so excited for you! Another doctor too!'

'Well, that's not really anything to do with it.' Susannah could feel her hackles rise like a cornered animal.

'No, but can you imagine, going from doctor's wife in the city to doctor's wife here, in your home village? A dog doctor! I mean, you couldn't write it better if you were a romance novelist.'

Susannah was well aware of the romance of it all, but the doctor's wife bit? That left her cold.

'He's not exactly like my ex, though. The two of them couldn't be any more different if they tried.' It was one of the many reasons she was attracted to Chris in the first place. 'Is that really what you think?'

They were in the office now, the floor covered to give them time to complete their paperwork for the incoming patients that week. They had to make sure that they were catering for their needs as best they could, making sure the rooms and equipment were ready to use and their individual care plans updated with all relevant information. Helen looked up, pen poised.

'Is what really what I think?'

Susannah played it down, but it had stung. Helen's comment had knocked her to her core, and now it was all she could think of. Was she repeating history? Was she destined to be a doctor's wife again, like before?

'That, you know, I have a "type".'

'Well, doesn't everyone? I know you've had it hard, but it wasn't all bad, was it? You were happy with him for a while.'

Susannah's face was scrunched up so tight she could barely speak.

'Helen, I barely survived the last time. We were happy, but that was because I didn't know who the hell I married.' It didn't matter that he was a doctor. She hadn't gone out and set her cap at him. He'd pursued her. They'd got on, he was good at work, easy to be around. She'd thought he was the one, and she'd changed herself to allow him to follow his dreams. And then, like a shifty pigeon, he'd gone and pooped all over the patio, full of the food she'd provided. It was a pretty rough analogy for a relationship ending. She was the one who'd got pooped on, and she wasn't about to offer herself up for more of the same. She realised Helen was staring at her open-mouthed, and she felt bad for a second. Helen's words had been a little close to the bone though. She'd been there; she knew what a toll it had taken on Susannah.

'Look, Hel, I—'

'No, I'm sorry. I didn't mean for it to come out that way.'

'It's fine. I need to go and check on Heather. Cover the floor?'

Helen knew she was being dismissed, and Susannah ignored her hurt look. She was butting in, and Susannah wanted to crawl away and inspect her wounds. She *never* liked to think of the good times with her ex, and Helen knew that too. It was getting too much, even for village life.

She wished she'd never started this whole dating thing. She knew Chris was wanting to take things slow—he hadn't said it, but it was obvious. He was still half in love with his wife, and grieving was like taming a monster. Monsters lurked in the shadows, and they came and went as they pleased. She'd grieved in her time. For patients, for their families. For her marriage. Being a divorcee was never on someone's life wish-list, after all. She was just mad that she had ignored the glaring signs that he wasn't the one. That he'd wanted *any*one, and his wife sitting at

home waiting for him. Now look at her. Five
minutes ago she'd been thinking about a future with Chris, now her armour was firmly
back on. She shuddered, and put on a brave
face before she entered Heather's room.

Heather Anderson was a stalwart of the
community, but her time was near now. Her
husband, Wilfred, had passed the year before, and Heather was pragmatic to say the
least. She had been one of Susannah's favourite neighbours growing up, and her own
parents had been friends of Heather's. She'd
seen Susannah grow up, and now Susannah
felt privileged that she could be there for her,
as her family and parents would have been if
they had been able.

Her soft tap on the door was unnecessary;
even at this hour Heather was up, watching
her favourite crime shows. She did love a box
set, and she didn't sleep much either.

'Hello, love.' Heather raised her hand to
usher her closer. Susannah took a seat close
to her, taking her hand and checking her vitals. She was comfortable, and pain free,
which was a good sign. 'You look bothered
by something.' She nodded towards the monitors. 'If it's that, don't you worry.' She smiled,
settling back down on the pillows. 'I'm fine.'

Susannah gently rubbed her finger along Heather's arm with her gloved hand.

'I know, I can see that. No pain?' A shake of the head.

'No, love, Wilf's waiting. I'm ready.'

'I know you are,' Susannah said softly. She'd said it before and Susannah knew it was the truth. She was tired, in mind and body. 'Can I do anything for you?'

Heather patted her hand, pausing the already muted TV. Gil Grissom stood frozen on the screen on the wall by her bed.

'You can tell me what's wrong. You don't look happy.'

Susannah rolled her eyes. 'I'm fine.'

Heather stared at her till she caved.

'It's nothing really. Dating has been a bit of a learning curve, and Helen just said something that's got me thinking.' She got on with the job of checking Heather's vitals, checking her charts and noting down her pain levels. 'So, you have some visitors coming, I hear?'

'Not till later. Go on, tell me what's wrong with this new man in your life.' Heather's eyes sparkled as she smiled at Susannah.

'Really? You really want to hear this?'

'Almost as much as I want Gil Grissom to come visit.'

Susannah smirked.

'Okay. She said something about being a doctor's wife again, and it just left me cold.'

'I bet it did. Tell me about him.'

'Chris? He's nice. He was a bit prickly at first, but he's widowed.' She bit her lip but the words were already out. 'Not that it's a bad thing, he's just…dealing with stuff, I guess. We keep clashing on things, and his temperament is a bit up and down.'

'Makes sense. I was a dragon when Wilf passed. So, he's the new village vet? That's great, isn't it? You love your dogs; it makes sense.'

'It does, and that's the problem, I think. John and I made sense at first, and this is my home. Imagine how awkward it will be when we break up? We're not even in a proper relationship yet and it's just so draining trying to work out what to do for the best.'

'Do you want to break up?'

'Well, no, and we're only dating.'

'That's like saying you are nearly a couple; it's the same thing if you're only seeing each other. Do you like him?'

'Yeah, but he is a doctor.'

'So?' Heather leaned forward, producing a flash of pain across her features. Susannah resisted the urge to run up and comfort her. She waited till Heather had settled

down again, checking her monitors whenever Heather wasn't looking. She didn't want
to take one ounce of dignity away from her
friend. It was ingrained in her nursing skills,
and Heather was a proud woman, illness be
damned. 'That's not why you like him, is it?'

'Oh, God, no. I met him at the practice,
and he was rude and all coiled up. I didn't
like him one bit.'

Heather said nothing, but she spoke vol-
umes with her expression. Susannah filled
the silence for her. 'But he's not like that really. He's all bluster, and he's so soft with
the animals. It's ridiculously cute. He's at my
house now, looking after a litter of puppies
he helped deliver.'

That got a reaction. 'So, Solitary Cottage
isn't so solitary any more, and you're freak-
ing out that you're repeating your past.'

'Yes!' Susannah prodded out with her finger. 'Exactly! And what if I am, and then I've
got another messy break-up and it's all played
out in front of the village?'

Heather shook her head. 'Listen to me,
John wasn't it, and there's no shame in that.
Divorces aren't what they used to be! Oh, if
they had been back in my day, lots of mar-
riages would have crumbled. Wilf and I were
lucky, but we had to work hard to keep it that

way. This village will see everything, I know that, but don't let it stop you.' She squeezed her hand, and Susannah's eyes brimmed with tears. 'Don't waste it. Your mum and dad would break their hearts if their little fireball wasn't happy.'

Susannah snorted through her tears. Her dad had always called her *fireball* because she had been a force of nature from the minute she could get around. The name had stuck within their little circle of friends. Heather was one of the last, and it saddened her more than she could ever let on.

'It sounds like they are two very different people. Having a medical degree doesn't make him a bad choice for you. I think you've already made up your mind what to do. All I can say is that everything you have done makes you the person you are, and I'm so proud of you. I know you'll be just fine.'

The two women wept together for a little while, till it descended into laughter. Susannah was soon back on the floor, her face back on, and she worked like a Trojan for the rest of her shift. It wasn't until she was on her way home that she realised Heather was right. She had made her mind up. She'd get through the meeting, and then speak to Chris. See once and for all what they had.

CHAPTER EIGHT

CHRIS'S ALARM WENT off on his phone, and
that was when things went downhill. His calendar notifications popped up on the screen,
and when he read them he felt sick. It was
such an innocuous reminder, but it felt as if
someone had stuck a scalpel straight through
his heart.

Anniversary—make arrangements

That was it. Hardly heartfelt, but it was
there. A remnant from a former life, but as
he was reading it in Susannah's spare room,
the timing felt all wrong. He'd thought he'd
deleted them all. He opened his calendar and
deleted it for ever. He sank back under the
covers, remembering when he'd put the reminder in his calendar in the first place. He'd
forgotten their second anniversary. They'd
both been so busy with work, but he had

blanked the whole thing. It had caused a row, but an empty one. She'd remembered just in time, but not enough in advance to get him a card either.

It should have shocked them, but it was just their life. He'd of course made an effort since, hating the feeling that something so special could be forgotten so fast, but it had been more of a perfunctory obligation written like that. He always kicked himself for how distracted he'd been, how distracted they'd *both* been. They'd been happy, but then when she'd become sick, their happiness in their careers had been all but on hold, and the void had been palpable without the work, and the noise, and the swanky nights out, and the scores of friends.

He'd missed most of his marriage.

The bit he missed the most was sharing a life with someone. He wasn't lonely per se, but reading that notification had made him think of all the other times he'd received little reminders that he'd had a life, and now he was trying to live another one. A more centred one. He'd spent three nights at Solitary Cottage now, and today, the anniversary, was the day of the charity-drive meeting with the volunteers. Bad timing, given that it would be the first public event in the village where he and Susannah would be together, on show. It felt like bad taste, but it was just business. He could get through the night and take her out later in the week. They had that shopping trip planned at the weekend—perhaps he could extend it to dinner too. It would be nice to spend more time with her.

He went to get dressed and see to the dogs. He had an early appointment, so he was leaving half an hour before she got back. Trudy was coming up to hold the fort and tonight she was taking the night shift for him as her daughter had begged to spend time with the puppies.

He'd not wanted to say no, but he was secretly gutted that he wouldn't be there longer. He quite liked being part of Susannah's world. They just needed to get the village meeting out of the way, get the event organised, and then they could focus on them. After Monday, things would be much easier.

'There's quite a lot of people out there,' Susannah murmured from the position behind the curtain. Her hands clasped around the velvet were shaking, sending little ripples all the way up the fabric. 'I didn't think so many people would come.'

'I know. I feel like Bon Jovi,' Chris said

beside her. He looked grumpy, as he had when they'd first met. 'Shall we just go out and get it over with?'

He wasn't looking at her, his gaze focused on the people through the gap in the curtain, so she didn't have to try to hide her hurt.

'Sure,' she said, clapping her hands together to keep them from smacking him around the face. 'If you're ready.'

He huffed in response, but she was already through the curtain and down the stage steps. She took a seat at the table at the front of the stage. What looked like the whole village was sitting in front of them, talking amongst themselves on the plastic chairs set out for the meeting. Hendrix was being fussed over by Cheryl, who was sitting with the other nurses on the front row. When Cheryl saw her, she motioned to everyone there and gave her an enthusiastic thumbs-up. Chris took his seat next to her and placed his hand on her lap— just for a moment, and then it was gone. She felt the heat from his body seep through her jeans. He was shuffling papers around on a clipboard now, looking both stern and official. She wanted to roll her eyes at him, but when she glanced back at the chairs, she knew that their every move was being watched. She almost wished that Heather could be here, just so she would see it. It really was something to marvel at. The residents of Puddle Lake, and their rather long bird-like necks, leaning close and sticking their metaphorical beaks into everything new and shiny.

She straightened her top, and called the meeting to order by standing up and introducing herself. The hall fell silent as she detailed her plans for the first ever charity drive being held in the grounds of Dr Jennings's home. Chris blushed when they applauded him, and she tried to catch his eye, but he was looking everywhere but her.

What's his deal?

His mood was making the doubts in her mind scream louder. Once the introduction had been done, the shelter teams all had their introductions to make, detailing their work and what they would need on the day. As the two of them sat at the top table, listening to the people come up and talk, the awkward feeling between them seemed to grow thicker around them. She put her hand on his knee, and he jumped. She snapped her hand back as if she'd been burned.

'What's wrong?' she whispered across to him, keeping an eye on the crowd for onlookers.

'Nothing,' he whispered back. 'Just trying to concentrate.' He leaned in closer to the front of the table, as if the extra half-inch would give him bat-like hearing. She started clicking her pen and heard him tut. 'Do you mind?'

She put the pen on the table with a clatter.

'Nope,' she said briskly. 'Not at all.' She stood up and headed to the refreshments table. There had been some wine donated for the meeting, to try to get the volunteers to be a little forthcoming with offers of help on the day. There was half a bottle of white left, and she drained the contents into the biggest glass she could see on the table before heading back to her seat. Chris was watching her return, and she waited for him to react to her. His face was pure stone. Expressionless. Giving nothing away. Solidly closed off from her. She'd drunk half the glass by the time her bottom hit the seat pad.

'Sorry. I just feel a little on show. It's been a bit of a weird day.'

She heard him, but she didn't acknowledge it. She focused on the meeting for the rest of the time, and then they were busy mingling, chatting to people about dogs they might be interested in, and introducing the shelter teams to the villagers that would be helping on the day. Before too long, they had a solid plan and she could see things start to take shape. The volunteers all had jobs before and on the day, and the rest were co-ordinating with each other. Chris had dealt with the legal side of the hosting duties, and Susannah had made sure medical, first aid and facilities were covered, and safety would be maintained on the day.

The dogs would be a little stressed if the schedule was too overwhelming, but by the looks on some of the faces of those in attendance this evening, the homeless hounds would be able to melt a heart or two. It was all coming together, but she just felt wretched about having had the idea in the first place. There was no getting out of this now, and as it was now being held in his grounds, it was even worse.

Once the last person left, and she and Chris were saying goodbye to the hall warden, she was desperate to get home.

'I am sorry, for earlier.'

Damn. Almost got to my car, too.

She turned and he was standing behind her, car keys in hand. She was hauling her handbag, her file for the charity drive, and a rather cumbersome portable pin board. Her keys were between her teeth. Reaching out an awkward hand, she dropped them into it and braced herself for an awkward chat. The contents of her arms suddenly felt a lot heavier.

'Sorry for what?'

Does he even know how mad I am at him? For being so aloof, when I was already having mixed feelings and swirling doubt. He doesn't see the doubts, and I know I can't blame him for something he knew nothing of, but...oh. It just shouldn't be this hard. I feel like I'm going to get hurt here. I need to protect myself. There's just too much baggage on both sides. We'll never be able to fit it all under one roof.

Helen's words were etched on her brain.

'Being a moody so-and-so.' He stepped closer and lifted the heavy board from her hands. 'It's been a weird day. I just wanted to get the meeting done.'

'I know, I get it. I do too, but these mood swings, Chris? I don't get them.' She turned to go to her car, clicking the doors open on the key and trying not to drop everything. He was there, right beside her, opening the boot.

'I know, and you don't have to get them. It's just a weird day, like I said. I needed to focus on work.'

Susannah put everything into the boot, taking the board from him and shoving it on top. She shut the door up and headed to the driver seat.

'Wait, Susie.'

'Susannah. I'm really tired, Chris. It's been a rough few days...my friend is...sick. Can we talk tomorrow?'

'I just wanted to say sorry.' His words were a little clipped. His jaw tensed when she focused her eyes on his. 'That's all. I know you've been busy, and I'm sorry about your friend. You know that. I just think we need to talk, soon. I can explain.'

And there it is. His opener or mine? Am I going to be dumped before I can get in first?

'We do need to talk.' She nodded, not looking away. 'I have some things I want to say.'

'Me too.' His face had brightened, but then he bit his lip. 'Just not today; I can't today. I have to work late tomorrow too—the surgery is offering some later sessions now. Some classes, things like that.' He was rambling now, and he looked flushed.

'Okay, later in the week is probably better anyway.'

'Saturday, then?'

Saturday? Something jangled in her memory, but it was wily. She couldn't quite remember. Her blank expression gave her away, and Chris straightened up a little taller.

'Er…yeah. Our shopping trip.'

'Oh, yes!' She slapped herself on the forehead, wanting the ground to swallow her up. Or better, for her to get in her car and drive home as fast as she could. 'I'm sorry! Er… yes, we could do that.' It would give her time to work out just what the hell she wanted to say to him. How she would be able to look him in the eye when they worked together. 'I'd better go.' She couldn't look him in the eye, so she knew that wasn't going to be easy.

'Susannah, look at me.'

She could barely hold her keys, she was so sweaty-handed. Gripping them tighter, she turned and leaned her back against the car door.

'Chris, I don't think I can do this.'

His jaw flexed.

'I know you're tired, but Saturday is a way off…'

'No.' She swallowed. 'I mean, I don't think I can do…this.' She pointed her finger between her and him. He took a step closer and she yanked her hand back before he could grasp it.

'Susie, I know I've been grumpy, but I really like you.'

'I really like you, but it's just not going to work.' She flexed her jaw to match his. 'I promised myself that I would never be second best again. We're already so in each other's lives, I just don't think it would end well. For either of us. Puddle Lake is a small place. People talk.'

'Screw the people.'

'What, all of them?' He didn't respond to her failed attempt at humour. He was mad, she realised. She could see it in his eyes.

'You know what I mean. I would never put you second best.'

'You're still grieving for your wife.'

She'd never said it out loud to him before, but she'd always known it. He was half consumed by it, but his grief was twisted around his gut, hidden from view to most people. Even himself, at times.

'That's not fair. Or strictly true.'

'Of course it is, Chris, and I don't blame you one bit. You should never feel bad for loving your wife.'

'It's not that. It's more than that.'

Susannah didn't want to hear him trying to explain something she understood only too well. She knew grief; it was a silent companion of hers. It had walked the hallways of the hospice many a time. Sometimes, she'd fallen into step right along with it.

'I just can't risk it again, I'm sorry.'

* * *

'Risk what again? Susannah, this is madness. Why are you walking away?'

'I'm tired!' she half shouted back at him. 'I'm tired of doing things for everyone else, and not expecting anything back. Okay? Spoiled princess, eh? My ex-husband treated me like I was an accessory to his life, and utterly disposable. Just like the poor dogs that I look after. I am sick and tired of people taking me—or anyone—for granted, and I just can't be in a relationship like that again.'

Chris was ashen, his mouth in a frozen grimace, his head turning from side, to side, to side.

'You've read this all wrong, Susie.'

'Are you grieving for your wife, yes or no?'

He crushed his lips together. 'It's not that simple. We were very different—'

'Please,' she half whispered. 'Just be honest.'

His eyes shuttered closed. 'Yes. Surely you don't judge me for that?'

'Of course I don't! I just mean that it's still too fresh, and with everything else…'

'Like what?' He wasn't getting it, and she wasn't explaining herself well either. She couldn't say everything she was feeling. One half of her wanted to tell herself to shut up, that the man in front of her was getting hurt by her words, and that was the last thing she'd wanted to do. The problem was, the other half of her, the one still smarting from the epic and messy divorce in her past, wanted to run back to her cottage, lock the door and never leave again. This was exactly what she'd feared.

'I don't know.' She shrugged weakly. His eyes flashed with frustration and she gabbled on to fill the silence, to stop him from saying something nice to change her mind. 'Lots of things. Your work is important to you, just like mine is.' He winced when she mentioned her job again, and she found the resolve she needed. 'See, you can't even stand me mentioning work! And with us working together, your wife, my ex-issues…it's just too much. I don't want to lose your friendship.'

He snorted at that. 'We were never just friends, Susie, and you know it.'

She looked at his chest, rising and falling rapidly. Was his heart racing as fast as hers? She could see Roz now, and Helen, being all sympathetic to her face but lamenting her love woes to each other when she wasn't there. They wouldn't be mean, but they wouldn't understand her reasons either. Her divorce had put her through the wringer too much already. She would not let Puddle Lake become a place she wanted to leave. Even if it meant pining for the vet from afar. It was safer that way at least.

'I just think it's the timing, Chris. I'm sorry.'

She looked straight at him, trying not to see the tight clench of his jaw, his beautiful eyes that were scanning her face urgently for any sign of a chink in her armour. She had opened her car door by the time he spoke again.

'So that's it? You've decided that it won't work, and that's that?'

She sat down in the driver seat, and when she went to close the door he didn't stop her. He just stood there, watching her pull her belt on and start the engine. She was about to put the car in gear when there was a tap at her window. She wound her window down but kept her eyes on the view in front of her.

'Susie, will you look at me?'

When their eyes locked, she felt the familiar pull of him. The jolt of electricity that ran through her when she looked into the eyes of the man she had once thought so bullish. They were marked with hurt now, and she shook her head.

'I'm sorry, Chris, but I really think it's for the best. I have to go.'

She managed to keep the tears at bay till he was out of sight. He didn't move when she drove away. She'd left him standing there, watching her leave. She couldn't take the look in his eyes, and when she wiped at her tears in the rear-view mirror, she saw the same reflected in her own watery globes.

When she got back to Solitary Cottage, she spent the night looking after the dogs, crying over her own cowardice and fear. Chris called her twice; each time she let it go to voicemail. The third time he tried, she turned it off altogether and shoved it into her nightstand.

Chris called again, and it went to voicemail without ringing once. He growled in frustration, throwing his phone onto the couch next to him. Hendrix jumped up from his bed, gripping the phone in his mouth and plonking it back on his lap, a string of dog spit now splatted across the screen. Chris rolled his eyes at the eager hound.

'Hendrix, I tried. She doesn't want to speak to me.' Nothing but a head tilt and a groan. 'Oh, come on, that's not fair. It's not my fault.' Hendrix lifted a paw and covered one of his eyes. 'It's not! She called it off.' Hendrix dropped his paw and jabbed the phone with his slender snout. 'Oh, come on, what makes you the dating expert? You don't even have testicles.' Hendrix omitted a low howl that made Chris cringe to the tips of his toes. 'Okay, sorry.' He leaned forward to stroke him, and Hendrix nuzzled into his hand. 'That was mean, and we both know I'm not really mean. Not that it matters now. She thinks I'm some damaged workaholic city boy.' Hendrix barked once, and Chris tilted his face to the side to match the dog's. 'Listen, I know you're not really talking to me, but that felt like a low blow. I'd say we're even now.' Reaching for his phone, he tapped out a message.

I hope you got home safe. I want to talk about this, I have things to say. Think about it?

He thought about adding a kiss, or even a funny dog emoji, but instead he slapped the silly thought away with a swift tap to the forehead. He deleted the message and threw the phone back into its original discarded spot. Hendrix groaned and headed to his bed. Moments later, a loud snore filled the room. Chris sighed heavily, reaching for the remote and putting the TV on. There was a vet show on, one of the good ones, and he watched the rather jolly vet on the screen explain what he was doing to the camera. His left arm was shoulder-deep in a rather bored-looking Holstein-Friesian cow, who was known on the farm as Mrs Butterfield, with a suspected prolapse. As he watched, he remembered a conversation he'd once had, back in his old home, on his old couch...

'This show again? That vet is far too happy sometimes.'

Chris chuckled, frowning as he turned and saw his wife's pale face.

'Are you okay? Warm enough?'

Karen rolled her eyes from under the layer of covers she was wrapped in.

'I'm like a blanket burrito. I'm warm enough, trust me.'

'You look a little pale. Do you want a drink?'

'I want you to stop fussing. You know what chemo's like.' He nodded grimly. He'd seen her go through it enough times to understand she was feeling ill. They watched TV for a while in silence. There were far too many silences between them now. It was as though they'd just run out of things to say. The things

they'd spoken of before didn't feature much in their lives any more. Karen pointed at the screen.

'That's what you should do.'

'We don't get many pigs at the practice, aside from the odd pot-bellied house pet.'

'No.' She reached for her water. Chris's hands itched to help the straw to her mouth, but he knew she would ask if she needed it. 'Open a practice in the country.'

Chris's head snapped to hers.

'That's not funny.'

'I'm not being funny.' The water she'd sipped went down the wrong hole, and she coughed. He went to help her, but she coughed again and held up a hand to stop him. 'I'm fine.' She wiped her mouth on one of her burrito blankets. 'Please stop fussing.'

'I'll stop fussing when you stop making bad jokes.'

'It's not a joke,' she retorted, smiling at him. 'I could see you doing that, living in the fresh air. Stress free.'

'He just got kicked in the knee by that goat; it hardly looks stress free. You hate the country anyway!'

'Well, that doesn't really matter, does it?'

His jaw clenched, and she smiled apologetically. You know what I mean.'

Chris reached for her hand, clasping it between his. 'I'll be fine. I love you so much.'

She squeezed his hand tight, and he moved it to his lips to bestow a soft kiss on her pale skin. 'You're a rubbish liar, you know that, right? I love you too,' she said, giving him the smile she always did. The smile he only saw when she gave it to him, and him alone. 'I just want you to enjoy your life. That's all I want for you. Please don't bury yourself in your work again.'

'I won't, I promise.'

He'd promised that to her often since that night, over and over every time she asked it of him. He'd done it too, not just to fulfil a promise, but the more she'd spoken about it, the more it hadn't seemed so alien to him after she'd passed. His old life had moved on and left him behind. He'd still failed though. What was it that Karen had said? Something about being happy. He was the village vet now, but he was lacking in the jolly part. He'd upped and moved, but then work had been his focus. He'd grown mean, and scrunched in on himself, like a tricky tumour, hiding between organs and tissues, throwing out its poison and not being touchable. Unreachable to the light, and hard to identify where work started and he ended.

Till Susannah had walked in, with the hound that was now snoring like a walrus beside him. They'd both bounded into his life, colourful and gleeful and optimistic. He'd felt irritated by her that day, incensed that someone could be that full of joy.

'She woke me up, you know,' he said to the dog. Hendrix retorted with a snuffle and a flick of his paw. He was probably after a dream rabbit. Maybe he was talking to the empty room. Maybe he was hoping Karen would hear him. As odd as it was, he knew what she would have said.

A promise is a promise.

It was what she'd always said, when he'd asked her to change the subject on LAH. Life after her. It had seemed so abstract at the time, like a child thinking about being their grandparents' age. Like something far away in the future. When the time had come, he'd turned on the autopilot. He'd got through the funeral; he'd tried to carry on as before. His old routines. Her words had come back into his mind so many times before he'd finally decided to go for it.

He'd been meant to come here—he knew that now. He wanted to be here. He liked his new life, and he was ready to share it again. The whole day had been a bust, the anniversary triggering his guilt. The guilt that he'd felt alone when he was sitting by Karen's bedside. The guilt that he'd put not his wife on a pedestal but work instead. Work didn't cuddle you after the loss of a patient. It didn't call to tell you it loved you. He'd chosen wrongly, and he'd tried so hard to make it up to Karen before she died. He'd chosen her, but it had been too late. Their time had already been cut short. Given an expiration date.

Second best. That was what Susannah had said to him. Her ex had neglected her too, in a different way. He'd strayed. Taken her for granted in his own cruel way. It was ironic really. He'd been half twisted with grief and guilt over not realising what he had, and she was too scared of him hurting her to realise that he would *never* do that to her. Work was important, yes, and he'd fallen back into his old ways that day to cope with the significance of the date. That was it, he realised. She'd seen a glimpse of the old him, and she'd had déjà vu. He wanted to kick himself for not realising sooner. Why did he never work things out till it was too late? He stood up off the couch, grabbing his phone and keys.

'Hendrix, I'm going out.'

As he pulled his car up to Solitary Cottage, his headlights picked up a flash of something brightly coloured coming out of the front door. He parked next to Susannah's car, pulling the handbrake on. He could hear keys jingling, and Susannah's voice, full of panic.

'I'm coming, okay? I just need to lock up.' She ended the call, shoving her phone into her coat pocket and cursing loudly as she dropped her keys.

'Susannah? You okay?'

She whirled around, and his heart missed a beat. She was crying, shaking, fumbling to find the right key on her chain.

'What are you doing here?'

'I came to— What's wrong?'

'My friend, in the hospice...' She dissolved into sobs once more, and shook her head, a look of anger crossing her face. She was mad at herself for being emotional. 'It's nearly time. I have to go.'

She turned and tried to lock her door again. Chris stepped forward, taking the keys from

her gently and locking up. She tried to take
the keys from him, but he held them back.

'You can't drive like this, Susie.' His heart
pumped when he realised what he needed to
do. 'I'll drive you to the hospice.'

Her jaw dropped even through her sobs,
but he'd already wrapped his arms around her
and steered her to his car. He got her inside,
and drove wordlessly to the hospice, listening as she called Roz back. Heather was asking for her. Chris reached for her free hand
with his. She didn't let go till they pulled up
outside.

'Thank you,' she said, distracted as she
left. 'I know this was hard for you.'

They were both standing at the front of the
car. Close enough to touch, but he didn't try.

'Anything for you.'

She smiled through her tears, and, stepping towards him, she stood on her tiptoes
and touched her lips to his. *Zolt!* He kissed
her back, pulling her close and wishing he
could tuck her into himself. To save her from
the pain she was in. She kissed him till he
tasted the salt of her tears, felt the tears on
his cheeks, his hands as they embraced.

'I won't forget this,' she whispered, leaning up for one last touch of his lips. 'You're
a good man.'

Then she was off, running towards the doors. He stood there for a while, touching his fingertips to his mouth and wiping away the evidence of her sobs, and then he turned to get back into the car.

Twenty minutes later, he was still there, standing at the doors to the hospice, willing his feet to move.

'Work, damn you!' he said to his un-cooperative feet. He paced up and down. 'Come on!'

He punched himself in the leg, as if to wake it up. 'Get in there, she needs you!'

He was still chuntering, taking steps forward and back, when the door opened. He noticed a woman watching him.

'Chris, is it?'

Embarrassed by what she might have observed, he nodded his head dumbly. 'Er... yes. Chris Jennings, pleased to meet you. Roz, is it?'

Her lips quirked. 'Yes, that's me. Can I help?'

'I don't think so.'

'You might be surprised. You coming in?'

'I'm still trying to decide,' he admitted. 'I want to.' He swallowed, and straightened himself up. 'My wife passed away in a hospice, back home. I...don't do well going down memory lane. Is Susannah okay, and your friend?'

Roz nodded. 'Bearing up. I'm sorry for your loss.'

'Thanks, it was a while ago now.'

'Doesn't make it any easier. I'll leave you to it. There's no shame in admitting defeat today. Susannah would never judge you for that.'

'I know, and that makes it worse. I can't even make it through a door. I don't know how you do what you do. Either of you. I lost one person in a place like this, and that was more than enough.' He ran his hands through his hair, trying to ground himself into the moment. 'I want to be there for her.'

'Well, you're here, so that's a start, right?'

There it was again, that look. Roz looked as if she was in on something that he wasn't aware of. He caught sight of the doors behind her, and his legs turned to jelly.

'Yeah, but a start of what? At the moment, it feels like a panic attack.' Roz leaned closer, but said nothing.

'Well, I think that's for you to decide.' A buzzer went off in her pocket, and she turned to leave. 'Cup of tea?' she asked over her shoulder, a brow raised in query. 'I can bring you one out, and a sandwich maybe. If

I come out and you're gone, I won't tell her you stayed.' She gave him a friendly smile, one that reminded him of Susannah. 'It's nice to put a face to the name.'

Chris's heart swelled. Susannah had been talking about him to her friends. Maybe all was not lost. If she was talking about him, she was thinking about him. As he was her. He knew he couldn't get her out of his mind, despite his best efforts. The chance that she might be feeling the same preoccupation that he was for her gave him a warm glow.

'Nice to meet you too.' He stepped forward, and held out his hand. She shook it, and when she went to walk back inside, he took a deep breath, and followed her over the threshold.

CHAPTER NINE

HEATHER PASSED AWAY peacefully mere hours later, Susannah and her friends by her side as she slowly took her last breath. Susannah managed to keep her tears in till she had kissed everyone goodbye, and it wasn't till she got into the break room that she allowed herself to feel it. She cried herself to sleep on the couch, and that was where Roz found her sometime later.

'Hey,' she said softly once Susannah's eyes opened. Both women could tell the other had been crying, and Roz sank down beside her as she sat up. Roz passed her one of the mugs in her hand. Susannah thanked her and took a deep gulp of coffee.

'I've called Erika to cover for me today. I can't concentrate enough on the job.'

Susannah squeezed her arm. 'Good call. I'm glad I have a day off, to be honest.' The two women sat and sipped at their drinks, feeling drained and sad. 'It doesn't get any easier, does it?'

Roz shook her head. 'No, it doesn't, but I take some peace in knowing that we do everything we can. This place...' She looked around her, at the wall of thank-you cards and messages from grateful families, the pictures of them sitting with their loved ones punctuating the heartfelt, tear-stained words they wrote. 'It's not just a place of endings for them. It's a place that makes an unbearable time bearable.'

She was so right. Susannah felt exactly the same. Heather's loved ones couldn't thank them enough, and she knew that Heather had been comfortable and in a place filled with love and care. They did make a difference, to everyone who passed through those doors. She found her mind wandering again to her other source of pain. The fact that she was newly single, having walked away from the vet who was grieving for his wife and falling for her. She knew he was falling; she could tell. She felt the same way, and that was the problem. It sounded crazy, them being so different, but she just knew in her gut that she had more feelings for him than she should have. If she allowed herself to fall...

It was too late, she knew that. She took another deep gulp of her coffee, sighing so hard she pushed all the air from her lungs. Roz misread her melancholy a little and wrapped her arm around her.

'She's free now, love. Heather was ready to go, bless her. Are you going to be okay? You can come to mine if you like; we can watch some rubbish daytime TV and eat some major carbs.'

'I wasn't thinking about Heather, not just about her anyway. I was thinking about Chris.'

'Oh, yeah? Well, that's good, isn't it?'

'Not really. I think we're done. Too many things against it, I think.'

His face last night... I bet there are gravel tracks up the drive from his quick getaway.

She'd just wanted him with her, but her job was coming between them again. She wanted to share her whole life with someone, but the fear in his face had haunted her, even at Heather's bedside. This was the job, or a huge part of it. Being there for people in the dark times gave her comfort; it fulfilled her even more than placing a foster dog. Could she really ever share that with him?

'Okay.' Roz's delayed reply distracted her from her own wishy-washy thoughts.

'Is that all you're going to say? Okay?'

'Well, you didn't give me much to go on.'

'Sorry. I'm tired. I don't think my decision-making skills are quite up to par.'

'I know, but that's never stopped you before. You got scared, didn't you? With the vet.'

She glared at her friend, but that only made Roz laugh. 'Oh, come on, I'm not evil. I've been a pushy so and so, maybe…'

'Definitely. And Helen.'

'Okay. I pushed because you needed it. Helen loves you too. I was just saying that I think you got scared! You changed when you met him.'

'I despised him when I met him.'

'No, you didn't. Not really.'

'Yes, I did. I wished every type of pox upon that man. I was livid!'

'Because you fancied him.'

'No—'

'Yes! He annoyed you, yes, but you have never talked so much about a man who you supposedly despised. You fancied him, and you were glad he was a massive idiot, because it scared you into thinking about dating again. That's what the app was about! To give you a shove.'

Susannah shook her head, but she was smiling. 'Am I really that stubborn? I really thought you and Helen were being cows, you know.'

They both giggled, and the tension that Susannah had been feeling around her fell away. She had read it wrong.

'Helen was really scared you were going to flip,' Roz confided with a titter. 'I had to convince her it would work, and that I'd take the rap. Heather was in on it.'

The two women fell silent when they re-alised her co-conspirator was no longer here to share the moment. Of course, they still felt her in the room.

'Well, thank you, Heather,' Susannah said to the ceiling. 'I flipped out on him though, spouted on about being second best.' She put her head in her hand. She could have fallen asleep right there and then. 'Oh, my God. And I talked about his wife too. I'm awful.'

'Hey! That's my friend you're talking about.'

She sat up, putting the now half-empty mug on the side. Coffee slopped onto the table. She mopped at it with the sleeve of her coat.

'I messed up, I think. We could have been friends, but I handled it wrong. I really like him, but I just can't go through it again. This might sound stupid, but I want the fairy tale,

I guess. You know? Someone who puts you first, and makes you feel loved?'

'That's not stupid. It's just far less easy to find in the real world than in a book. It's no coincidence so many women read those books you love. They want the same. Everyone wants to be cherished, Suze. It's human nature.'

'He reminds me of John sometimes. He'll feel something, and then it's all locked up again. Like he found a leak in his heart and plugged it quick. John did the same, and he just buried himself so deeply in work he never came out the same. Geez, I'm here moaning, and Heather... I just think it's best if we stay apart for a bit, till I can get my feelings sorted out.' She didn't even sound as if she meant it to her own ears. She looked to see if her friend had bought it. Roz said nothing, but she had that look about her. The one that meant she was fooling no one. 'Spill it. I know you have something to say.'

Roz pretended to look surprised, but Susannah raised a brow and she crumpled like a cheap suit.

'I think you read him wrong, to be honest. He's here. I put him up on a cot in one of the family rooms.'

Susannah laughed. 'Very funny. He wouldn't set foot in this place.'

Roz squeezed her friend tight. 'You are dense sometimes. He never left the car park. I found him standing outside. He wanted to be here, for you. That's not putting someone second best in my book.'

Susannah had so many questions.

'Which family room?' was the one that burst from her mouth.

He was fast asleep, sprawled on the sofa with one hand over his face. The blanket he was under was half on the floor, and she bent to straighten it up. As she covered him, he awoke. He looked tired, drawn. She wondered how long he'd been sleeping.

'Hey,' he murmured. He sat up and motioned for her to sit next to him. She sat, and he pushed the blanket aside. 'Can I do anything to help?'

She smiled. 'No, but thanks for asking. She passed peacefully. Thanks for bringing me too. You were right; I wasn't in a fit state.' He didn't reply. 'You didn't need to stay.'

'Roz put me up. She's a character, isn't she?'

Susannah nodded, laughing despite her exhausted state. 'Yep, she's one of a kind all right. I can't believe you're here.'

He stood slowly, stretching out his limbs and tapping his foot on the floor as he walked around the room. He looked dishevelled, crumpled and utterly adorable. She was about to embrace him, to thank him for being there for her, but something stopped her. It was the look on his face. He was looking around the room as if he was looking for a rip cord somewhere.

'Neither can I. I almost vomited in the bushes at one point. Listen, I have to get back to the surgery, but I just wanted to be here.' His eyes inspected the room once more, and she wondered what he was seeing. What was going through his mind? He'd put himself through a night there, for her. The thought made her heart soar, but it brought something else into crystal clarity. Life was evil like that, sometimes.

His eyes zeroed in on hers, but she could tell he wasn't fully with her. He'd tried so hard, but he wasn't there yet. Would he ever be there? She played every scenario over and over in her head. Her work with the shelters and the dogs, her seeing him all the time at the surgery. She was in his life, she knew his colleagues, his patients even.

'Are you okay?' she made herself ask him, and she begged for the answer to be that he was healed. That he'd conquered a demon. 'I know last night must have been hard for you.' She wanted to say more, to tell him how much it had meant. *Everything.* He'd put her first, even over his own pain. She knew the cost was dear to him. When his eyes locked with hers, she knew it was too much.

She knew she was begging the Almighty for something impossible, but she held her breath and willed it into being anyway, with everything she had. They couldn't do this now. They were so close to...to...

'I'm fine.' He yawned, checking the clock. He rubbed her shoulder softly. 'I should go though. I'm sorry to leave you like this.' He was up and halfway across the room before she could blink. 'Do you need a lift?'

'No, thanks. Roz's here. Chris—'

'You don't have to thank me, Susie. We're friends, right? I wanted to help.' He smiled, but when she searched his eyes, they looked right through her. 'I'm really sorry about Heather. Look after yourself today.' He was looking at her as if she were a chipped china doll. His forehead was shiny with sweat, and his eyes kept finding the clock. 'I'll call you later, okay?'

He leaned in for a kiss, but she turned so he got her cheek instead. He stilled for a moment, his lips meeting her forehead this time. She didn't dodge that one; she closed her eyes and cherished it. All the moments weren't nearly enough, and now there would be no more.

'It did mean a lot, you coming,' she said. She'd waited like a chicken for him to get to the door before she spoke. 'You don't have to worry about me though. Thanks for being a friend.'

She looked down at the floor, at the spot on the tile she'd planned to search for before she spoke. She knew her head wouldn't move an inch till he'd left. She couldn't take his face. Relief or disappointment would have crushed her to see on the face of the man she loved. 'I will always worry about you,' she heard him say.

The door closed behind him with a click.

'Well,' she said to herself, long after her vision had turned the spot on the floor to two blurry ones and his steps had faded away. 'Looks like that's that.'

CHAPTER TEN

EVEN IN PUDDLE LAKE, time didn't stand still.
Days turned into weeks. The season changed,
bringing with it the sunnier weather. Heather's funeral had taken place, and life was
moving on as it did. People went about their
days, and Susannah's life fell into the old
pattern of work and her dogs. The puppies
were nearly ready for homing now. Tank was
the liveliest of the bunch, and he kept her on
her toes when she was at home. The name
Chris had bestowed on him had stuck, and
he certainly lived up to it. She found herself wanting to send him pictures, but she
always stopped herself. He'd been at the
funeral—she'd seen him sitting at the back—
but when she'd gone to find him at the wake,
Cheryl had told her he'd been called away
on an emergency. It was the same when she
visited the practice. The times when they did

cross paths, they didn't speak much other than about the dogs, or the charity drive.

The drive was well under way now, the villagers all pulling their weight in their own ways. The pub had agreed to allow access to their toilets and were opening up their beer garden for the visitors. The local shops were all on board, advertising the event in their windows and donating prizes to the raffles. The hospice volunteers and crafty clan were working away, their knitting needles warm from all the things they were making. At one point there was a cotton shortage in the village, and the local craft shop was practically stripped bare. Everyone had gone all out, and Hendrix and Chris were one of the star attractions on the day. He was everywhere and nowhere in the village, like a will-o'-the-wisp. Now that there was a week to the event, the time had come to have another meeting. This time, at the venue itself: Chris's house.

She'd left work a little earlier that day. Trudy was on dog duty for her, and she wanted to be prepared for the meeting as best she could. It was one thing him keeping his distance but being at his house wasn't going to be easy if they were barely speaking. She was just getting into the car when she spotted what looked like Chris's car pulling in. He drove through the staff car park, heading round the building to where the visitors kept their cars. .

'That's weird,' she mumbled. She waited for him to come to the front door, but there was no sign. She gave it another ten minutes, and then dismissed it in her head. She was imagining things now. She thought she'd seen him there the other day too, in the corridor, but when she'd finished with her patient and gone back to check, there had been no one there. 'You're hallucinating, woman,' she said out loud. She started her car and headed for home. The sooner she got over this, the better.

'Do you think we've got enough nibbles?'

Hendrix was sitting at the foot of the table, licking his lips. He'd already swiped half a pork pie off the order from the butcher when Chris wasn't looking so he was in the doghouse. Hendrix woofed once.

'Yeah, that's what I thought. I did too much, didn't I?'

He'd been on tenterhooks all day waiting for the meeting. Half of Puddle Lake was descending on his house, many of whom remembered the past vet living there. The other half, the non-attending half, would no doubt be fully regaled of the evening's events. He'd never been so nervous in his life. He normally didn't really care what people thought; after all, he'd spent the last few months being the worst version of himself. Now, he wanted to fit in here. He wanted to help Susannah. He might have screwed things up when he first arrived, but he was changing.

His world wasn't devoid of joy any more. Sometimes, when he woke alone in his bed, the old feelings of despair would be there, right behind his eyes, and he'd have to resist the urge to pull his head under the covers and stay there. This morning, Hendrix had awoken him by jumping on his torso like a kid on a bouncy castle. His first moment had been laughter, and company. Watching the hound eyeing the food as if he was planning his next theft attempt, Chris couldn't help but smile. In the last few weeks, he'd made himself go out. He wanted to heal himself and give Susannah time to grieve for her friend. He knew she'd be there for everyone else, and he wanted to work on himself. For her and him. He'd forced himself to see the village as she did.

Walking the dogs, he'd met more locals and their hounds. Mrs Chan had brought a pineapple upside-down cake into the surgery. A sugar-free version, to thank him for Gustav's new vigour. The now rather slender cat could not only lick his man parts, but he was out terrorising the local mouse population like a sprightly kitten. She'd even brought a fat-free treat bag for Hendrix.

The villagers were slowly coming around to him, but he still didn't have the one person he wanted. Susannah was like a ghost now. He avoided her at the practice when he could, wanting to give her space. She didn't ask Cheryl about him, and his loyal receptionist was very quiet on the subject. Loyal to Susannah, probably.

Heather's funeral had been a real event. Quite different from the ones seared into his memory. The church had been full of colour, and Susannah the brightest one in the crowd. He'd stayed in the back, watching her take care of everyone around her. When she'd gone to the pulpit to say a few words, there had been no sadness in her tone. She'd spoken of Heather, to Heather. She'd shared memories that had the villagers rolling with laughter. The whole church had seemed to fill with love, and joy, and Chris had been amazed by her all over again. He couldn't imagine one person looking at her and making her second best. He wished he could meet her ex-husband, to tell him what an idiot he'd been.

It was hypocritical, in a way, he mused. He'd taken his wife for granted too. They'd both been guilty of that. It was the way of modern life, he thought. Moving here, meeting Susannah and the other people who lived their lives so differently, he felt as if he'd finally woken up. There was more to life than work, as rewarding as it was. Hendrix shared his life, his home, and quite often his bed. Even the dog he'd taken in knew the value of life better than the city version of himself had. He had a big house, a good salary, a thriving practice. None of that had altered, but it wasn't what he measured his achievements against any longer. His old friends had happily let him slink off, uncomfortable in the presence of such reality. Money couldn't cheat death, and being reminded of their own mortality had caused them to retreat, just as he had from them.

Sitting in the church that day, he'd seen it all. People laughing at memories they'd shared, holding each other as they cried. Being a supporting arm to a sobbing woman. A mother holding her child that bit closer.

Susannah, standing with the other nurses, saying goodbye to the friend they had loved and cared for till the end.

He wanted this life, more than anything. He wanted the colour, and the fresh air. He wanted to be mourned when he died, by a church full of people who knew and loved him. People he'd helped along the way. He wanted to be Mr Rogers, damn it. He wanted to be the person that Susannah deserved. He'd known that day that he'd fallen for her. Watching her speak of her friend, not shedding a tear or letting her voice waver, he'd longed to walk to the front of the church and throw his arms around her. He'd been so close, that night he'd driven to tell her how he felt. He'd been so close to telling her how she'd started to heal his closed-off, gnarled and battle-scarred heart, but he'd missed his chance. He couldn't do it now. At first she was grieving, and then time moved on and she still kept her distance. When they were in the same room, she was kind and polite. Friendly.

'I hope we can be friends,' she had said.

Yeah, that hit like a ton of bricks. Were we ever friends, really?

She'd cited his grief, but his wife was gone.

He had loved her, yes, but his grief was about the life he'd had as much as the person he'd lost.

The life he didn't fit into any more. The one he didn't miss now. He was the village vet, Puddle Lake was his home, and now he needed the woman to go with it. The new love he'd never thought to look for. The rainbow to his rain cloud. The light to his dark. Hell, he'd even stepped through the hospice doors for her. To be there, in case she needed him. When Roz had found him in the car park tying himself in knots, she'd given him the choice to go in with her, and he'd not even questioned it once his feet had finally moved forward. His hands had been shaking as he'd pushed open the foyer doors, and he'd waited for something to trigger his memories. A disinfectant smell, a poster on the wall. The beeps of the machines. There had been nothing. The minute he'd stepped in, all he'd seen was her. The place was a cacophony of colours too, the warmth of the painted walls filled with quirky art. There were no banal *Live, Laugh, Love* slogans to be seen. The whole place was built like the embrace of a loved one.

'Hang in there,' Roz had said to him as she showed him to one of the empty family rooms. 'Don't give up on her yet, okay? Heather is special to her. Her mother's best friend. It's a bit like losing her parents all over again, I think. Her work means such a lot to her.' She had given him a warm smile and patted him on the shoulder. 'Just hang in there, okay? You're good for her.'

She'd meant the words kindly, but they had hit like shrapnel. Ripping into him and leaving him bloody and shell-shocked.

You're good for her.

Am I?

He'd played those words over and over in his mind, and he didn't like the conclusion his tired brain kept coming to. He wasn't good for her, because if he were, wouldn't they be together now? He'd been mean to her since the minute he'd arrived, his anger and unprocessed feelings coiled around him like the bars of a prison. She was light, and caring, and happy. He'd dulled her light. He'd made her feel second best. He'd done it without meaning to, but it still stunned him. He didn't want to make the same mistakes all over again. He wanted to share a life with her, not have her on the periphery of friends, and possessions, and working every hour as though racing to some impossible goalpost that he would never reach anyway. Her friend had just passed away before her eyes, and when she'd come to the family room to find him, he'd walked away.

He'd had to get out of that room. When he'd known she was suffering, and going through that process just a few rooms away, it was all he had focused on. Being near her had felt so important, even if he couldn't be by her side to comfort her properly. She wasn't his, so that wasn't his place. He'd ignored the smells, the memories prickling at the corners of his brain. He'd coped, till he saw her.

She had looked so broken and sad. So tired. He'd known the nurse in her would feel relief for her friend, that the pain and the suffering had passed. He'd felt it too, and that was when the walls had started to close in around him. The smell had become noticeable once more.

He'd seen the hurt on her face, but he'd known in that moment he couldn't give her what she needed. What she deserved. Not quite yet. He hadn't been ready.

The day after, he'd called Roz, and now here they were. He'd thrown himself into village life. He'd bonded with his patients and their owners, he'd been seen out at events and eating in the café. Sitting in the pub beer garden after a long walk with Hendrix, chatting to the other pubgoers and swopping dog stories. He'd made an effort and, to his surprise, he'd actually enjoyed every minute of it. Even going to the hospice had exorcised some of his demons. Roz had helped him there too, allowing him to read to some of the lonelier patients when Susannah was out of sight. Many families still needed to keep the wolf from the door, even when their loved ones were sick. He'd filled in for them, reading books out loud, and playing cards in the games room. He'd even suggested that a therapy animal might be something to look into for some of the people who came through the doors.

He'd felt her presence on those corridors too. The place smelled like her. He could see first-hand how much the people in her life thought of her. She wasn't second best to anyone, and he needed her to see that.

They were now mere days away from the charity drive, and it had to go to plan. He wanted to do this day for her, host it in his house, show her *and* the village the real him. The new Chris, who cared, who wore his heart on his sleeve. It had to work. After the drive was done, the opportunity would be lost. She'd sent Trudy the last time she'd needed a vet for one of her rescues, and it was obvious that Trudy was well aware of their situation, as diplomatic as she was. He needed to get this right, and he needed every bit of help he could get.

The doorbell rang, and Hendrix bounded to the door, his nails click-clacking on the wooden floor as he jumped up at the door. Roz, Helen and Cheryl were all standing there, looking a little like the Sanderson Sisters, furtively looking around them for onlookers.

'Come in, ladies, thanks for coming. I really need your help.' He moved aside for them to come in, grabbing some of the bags of goodies they'd brought for the drive. Roz and Helen asked where the kitchen was, and hurried off. Cheryl loitered behind a little, and then surprised Chris by reaching out to hug him.

'Oh,' Chris said, surprised. He hugged her back. 'What's this for? Being a good boss?'

Cheryl pulled back laughing, picking a bit of dog hair off his shirt.

'That, and you finally asking for help. Honestly, Chris, I never thought you'd get it together.' She eyed him up and down. 'Well, you look smart. Are you sure you're ready for this?'

Chris thought of everything that had brought him to this day. To this village, to this practice, to Susannah and her army of amazing friends. These women would do anything for her, and he knew that feeling very well. It had consumed him for weeks.

'Not even a little bit, but I'm done with letting life happen. Are you sure you're ready? She'll be mad, you know.'

Roz cackled from behind them, Helen joining in.

'Oh, Christopher, you have no idea. She'll be livid! Which is precisely why you need to do it. It's perfect, Chris. Trust us.'

Chris laughed, looking at the three friends he'd come to know quite well. He could see why Susannah loved them.

'I do, ladies. Come on, we don't have long. Everyone else is briefed—do they know to keep schtum?'

'We natives can hold our own water, you know.' Helen was grinning at him now, patting Hendrix, who had decided that she was the one that would give him the most fuss. 'Can't we, Hendy?'

Roz chuckled, and Helen rolled her eyes at her.

'Okay, we all live in each other's pockets, but they won't spoil it—don't worry. They know what's important. You should see the sign-up sheet; it's going to be amazing!'

'I know. I still can't believe you came up with it.' That was from Cheryl, who was busy setting up a flipchart in the corner of the dining room.

'Thanks. I'm not that much of a bore, surely?'

The three women looked at each other, and he could tell that they were deciding how diplomatic they should be.

'Oh, come on! I know I was awful when I first came.'

'Mrs Chan was talking about getting a petition together to run you out of the village at one point. She said you were too political and curt.'

'Her cat was overweight—a petition wouldn't have sorted that,' he retorted huffily. Cheryl's lips clamped together, and she went red. He side-eyed her. 'You know I'm right.' She shook her head, but she was laughing.

'I'll give you that. Bygones, eh?'

The doorbell went, and all four of them jumped.

'Ready?' Chris asked. 'Not a word.'

The three women were now poised for action. For a second he felt like Charlie did when he had his angels in tow.

'We're ready.'

'What? Why are they here?'

Susannah jerked up the handbrake on her car and stared at the familiar vehicles that were parked outside Chris's house. Roz, Helen and Cheryl were already here? They'd not said anything to her. What was going on lately? Chris seemed to be everywhere these days; all she heard about was the kind village vet and his funny dog. *Her* funny dog, she thought childishly. *She'd* named him; *she'd* nursed him back to health. Now he was some kind of doggy celebrity, and everyone was singing his praises from Puddle Lake church to the outskirts of the village. Irony was a cruel mistress sometimes. When she'd liked Chris, the village hadn't and now, when she needed to keep her distance, it seemed as though the village had adopted him like a lucky stray.

'God, you sound bitter.' She was talking to herself in the mirror again, which only proved how bothered she was. It made it all the harder for her to keep her distance. He seemed better though, happier even. He was out and about, living his life. She was happy for him. She could lie to herself in the mirror all day long about how much of a chicken she felt for cutting loose before things really got started but she couldn't quite pull off deceiving herself about her feelings for him. She'd fallen for him, white coat and all, and she was miserable. She'd even told the shelter she wanted to keep Tank. She couldn't bear to let go of the dog he'd saved and named. Pathetic? Maybe, but Tank was staying put and that was that. She'd already taken him off the list of prospective dogs for the charity day.

The door opened before she even got to the front pathway.

'Oh, hey!' Roz exclaimed, heading out with Helen. 'You're early.' She passed something behind her back to Helen, who headed off to her car. Susannah didn't even register the movement.

'Er...yeah.' She checked her watch, even though she knew damn well what time it was. 'I got off early for once.' Roz nodded, but she was acting off. 'How come you're early?'

'Oh, Helen and I have something on tonight.' She was already retreating to her car, Helen already driving off with a wave. 'We'd better get off, see you at work!'

'Roz, wait...where...' Roz's car door shut with a click, and her engine roared into life

'…are you both going?' she said to the re-treating car. Roz held up a hand to wave goodbye, and she was gone.

Susannah got her phone out to ring her but, tutting, she put it back in her pocket. She had been a bit of a cow lately. It was no wonder her friends were not in a mood to stop and chat. Seemingly, the nicer and more sociable Chris got, the more she went the other way. Come to think of it, the people she had seen in the village lately had been a bit standoffish too. She looked at her drawn expression in the mirror, and, with a deep sigh, she slapped on some lippy and headed to the house. She was almost to the doors, when the other vil-lagers started arriving, taking with them the chance of any alone time with Chris. She had the dogs to get back to, and her foster cover to relieve.

Before she knew it, she was back home with the puppies and the minutiae of her daily life. Giving Tank an extra kiss before she headed to bed, she wondered why every-one around her was acting so weird. Maybe it was just her. Not being Miss Little Sunshine for once had been out of character for her, but she couldn't help it. She could feel the green-eyed monster pipe up at times too. Stupid re-ally, but it did tick her off. Right when she'd decided to be a grump, the once-hated village vet had transformed himself into a pillar of the community. This time next year he'd be a national treasure, and she'd be one of those women who got videotaped losing their temper in traffic and going viral for being a 'Karen' meme, whatever that meant If she wasn't so confused by the whole thing, she'd probably get a kick out of it.

CHAPTER ELEVEN

WHEN DAWN BROKE on the morning of the charity drive, Susannah opened her bedroom curtains and squinted at the first rays of sun. It was a beautiful summer's day, the ground dry and firm. Perfect conditions for an outdoor charity drive. She could scarcely believe it was here. Turning away from the window, she felt Tank nuzzle against her feet. She picked up the rambunctious puppy, who was still chewing on one of her fluffy white monogrammed slippers. She went to take it out of his mouth.

'Leave, Tank. Got out of your pen again, I see.' The stocky little puppy released the slipper, and a small trail of slobber slid from the mangled fabric, down the sleeve of her nightshirt. 'Ugh.' She gave it back to him. 'Ah well, guess these are yours now. Just leave my wellies and pumps alone. Do we have a deal?' The little puppy was already eviscerating the slipper again. She kissed his broad little face and set him down in his basket under the radiator. 'Trudy will come get you later, okay? I'll see you up there.'

The morning went even faster than Susannah had expected, and before she knew it, people were heading up to Chris's with their stalls and wares in boxes. Trudy and her daughter were on their way to collect some of the dogs at the cottage. There were three at her place ready to home, a Westie called Ricky, a beagle called Dynamo, and a rather nervous Yorkie called Neville. She had high hopes that these dogs, and many others from the shelters, would get a home today. It was what the whole thing had been for, and Susannah was hopeful it would all come off without a hitch.

As she drove through the village, her boot full of stuff for the day, she saw scores of people walking or driving up to Chris's house. When she turned the corner onto his property, she was taken aback to see all the activity. The place was crawling with people. The shelter vans were all there, setting up their areas for the dog shows and the meet-and-greet tents for prospective owners to bond with their possible new fur babies; the stalls were all around the front of the house, running like a ribbon the whole way around it.

'Wow,' she breathed, taking it in. She could scarcely believe the day had arrived, but here it was, looking even better than her wildest dreams. She pulled into a space in the trees, and, getting everything out of her car, she got to work.

'Morning!' Mrs Chan trilled, walking past her with a couple of cake tins stacked up. 'Doesn't it look great? You've done so well.'

'Thanks.' She smiled. 'It takes a village, right?' Mrs Chan laughed with her.

Everyone was bustling around inside, Hendrix barking at everyone from his position at the living-room window. Chris had obviously rather wisely decided to keep him away from the bustle. And, knowing the Doberman as she did, away from the food too. He'd once wolfed down a large pack of mince that had been defrosting on her sideboard. One that she had been planning to cook up for the dogs anyway. She laughed at the memory.

Heading straight down the side of the house, she stopped dead in her tracks. If the front was more than she'd expected, then the back gardens were like stepping into paradise. Everything was fantastic, and just as they'd planned it. There was a large area for the dog show, with obstacles in place in the centre. It looked amazing. She headed over with her piles of stuff, making a beeline for the hospice stall areas first. Everyone was in very high spirits, and raring to go.

'Hi! Almost time!' Helen was sitting at the information stand, ready to get people to donate via a regular monthly direct-debit payment, or give what they could as a one-off. 'It's really come together, hasn't it? Roz is over the moon.'

'Where is Roz?' Susannah asked, but Helen appeared not to hear her. She dropped off the supplies and checked in with the shelters. They all had information boards about the dogs, with some of the more sociable and less nervous ones there, ready to wag their tails and charm their way into a new life. She spent the next hour weaving around, making sure everything was on track and accounted for. Chris was nowhere to be seen, but she knew that he was running a tent for the practice, and would no doubt be busy. She looked around for Cheryl and Roz again, but, without finding them, she resumed her clipboard full of things to check off. She'd see them soon enough.

* * *

The day went so fast, and the crowds of people that showed up could have filled the village twice over. People were laughing, having fun on the tombola stalls and the games. The local radio station had come, and they were plugging the event for them, interviewing visitors and the shelter staff, talking about the dogs, and the hospice, and why they were all there, pulling together. The dog show had been a resounding success, and Hendrix had picked up an award for completing the circuit in record time. Cheryl had run him around the event, and Susannah found her mind wandering once more to their host as she listened to the DJ make another announcement.

'So, folks, as we know, the day has been great so far! People are digging deep for these charities, and, at the last count, we have made matches for over twenty dogs!'

Susannah, sitting on a camping chair at the corner of the fenced-off green, clapped, whistling with her fingers. Twenty dogs in just a few short hours! It was working. She felt the relief overcome her, and she wiped a tear from her cheek as she hollered with the rest of the applauding crowd. *Chris.* She looked for him in the crowd again, but he wasn't there. In the corner of her eye, she suddenly spotted Cheryl pulling out a large square object on a set of wheels. Neville from Oak Farm, complete with some fresh-looking hair implants, was helping her. A couple of women in the crowd giggled and waved to him.

Good for you, Nev. He does look good. More happy, confident.

He pushed the large object, which was covered in a sheet, into the centre of the field and winked at the ladies as he made his way back to the crowds. Susannah was just wondering what the heck the box was for, when her world went dark.

'Hey!' she shouted, but someone clamped a hand down over her mouth.

'Shush, it's me,' Roz said into her ear. She tied something round the back of Susannah's head, and she found herself being dragged off. Another set of arms reached for her, and she kicked out.

'Ow!' Cheryl cried out.

'Cheryl? Roz? Get this off me now! Argh!' She was silenced again, and felt her feet leave the floor. Her bottom was plonked into a rather hard chair, and then the hands were gone. She reached forward, trying to grab at them, but her hands hit something hard. *A wall?* She tried to stand, but then she heard Roz's voice over the microphone.

'What did you do?' Susannah growled under her breath. She tried to get the blindfold off, but felt someone slap her hand away. When she tried to turn around, realising that the walls were only on three sides, she was shoved back into her chair. 'When I get my hands on you, Cheryl, it's not going to be pretty. What are you doing?'

Roz's voice was booming across the crowd, the odd ripple of applause from the crowds erupting when she named and thanked the various people in attendance. Susannah folded her arms, and glowered beneath her blindfold.

'And now,' Roz said theatrically, 'we have a very special guest, with a very special surprise event! Can you put your hands together, please, for our host, our very own village vet, Dr Christopher Jennings?'

The crowd whooped even louder than the other times, and Susannah swore she heard Mrs Chan shout, 'That's my boy! Go, Chris!'

'Yay, Christopher!' she whooped along sarcastically. 'Jennings for mayor!' She held both hands up and waved tiny imaginary flags in his honour. 'Woo-hoo,' she mono-toned. *Kill me now.* That one was just for her.

'Thank you.' Chris spoke into the micro-phone now, and the crowd hushed. She could hear Hendrix bark, and he sounded close. 'And thank you, Puddle Lake, for giving me such a warm welcome to the village. I am only too happy to offer mine to you all today, and we're here now to celebrate one special lady. Cheryl, can you do the honours?'

Susannah felt Cheryl tug at the fabric at the back of her head, and she dug her nails into the soft flesh. Cheryl jumped back. 'Hey! Knock it off.'

'Knock it off? What's going on?'

'Trust me,' Cheryl said, right into her ear. Susannah sighed heavily but put her talons away. 'And get a manicure too. Geez.'

Susannah chuckled. 'I hope I drew blood. I'd better not be on a dunking stool. I mean it!' Cheryl just laughed, smoothing her hair down and retreating.

'Oh, it's much better than that. Hold tight!'

There was a series of bangs around her, and the blindfold fell away. Susannah opened her eyes, and the whole village was staring at her. The 'walls' she'd been beating against were gone, leaving only a wooden frame.

There was a sign at the front of the structure, but from her position she couldn't read what it said. She was still taking in her surroundings when Chris spoke again, and her eyes were on nothing but him.

He looked so handsome, so…peaceful. He was wearing an open-neck white shirt, a pair of dark blue jeans with wellies on. His hair was ruffled, and she knew he'd run his hands through it many times that day. Hendrix was sitting by him. She felt the old flicker of attraction burn in her chest. He walked over to her slowly, and, when he was close, he gave her a wink. The movement was so intimate, in front of the world, so sexy, that she was suddenly glad she'd been shoved onto a chair.

'Nothing that we see before us today would have been possible without our resident nurse and dog rescuer, Susannah Harkin. Now, if you don't know Susannah, she's pretty easy to spot. She dresses like Joseph in her Technicolor clothes, and she gives her heart and soul to this village, and to the people in it. I've never met a woman like her, and personally I'm very grateful that she crashed into my surgery one day, with this little monster in tow.' He nodded to Hendrix, who barked loudly, delighted to be mentioned. The crowd laughed along with Chris. 'I'm sure it's not a secret that when I first came, I was a little… sullen.'

Mrs Chan piped up. 'Understatement of the century!'

Chris threw her a wry look, his gorgeous brow raised, and Mrs Chan blew him a kiss. The crowd whooped.

'Yes, thank you, Mrs Chan. Well, I was a little lost when I first came here. Susannah was the one who made me realise just how much life has to offer, especially in this corner of the Earth. So I wanted to honour Susannah, and everything she does for her patients, her dear friends, and the animals she works with. I am sure you can all agree, and know even more than I do, that without her this village would not be quite as bright.'

His eyes were burning into hers now, and she looked right back at him. She couldn't tear her eyes away. 'What people might not know about Susannah is her love of romance novels, and how she loves matchmaking those gorgeous dogs with their new owners. So in honour of the day, and in the spirit of matchmaking…' Susannah groaned, and a ripple of laughter burbled around her '…what better way to honour her than to have our very own…' he pulled a sheet of cardboard she hadn't seen from the sign '… Village Matchmaker?'

The crowd gasped, applauded and whooped as he bent to take a bow at her feet. When he raised his gaze, her look of shock didn't seem to register with him. He flashed her a devilish look.

'The rules of the Matchmaker are simple: a person looking for a match signs up to see if they can find their match from the suitors in the audience!' He did a little gameshow host sweep of his hands, before cupping his mouth around the microphone. 'Keep it clean—we have animals and children present.' The crowd rippled with laughter, and Susannah was glued to the edge of her seat. Any trace of surly Chris was gone from the man she was observing.

'So, before we get started with our lucky contestants, starting with our resident and newly single farmer—give us a shout, Neville!' He turned in Neville's direction, and Neville stood from his seat, flexing his muscles and making the females in the crowd all catcall loudly. Susannah spotted his ex-wife, sitting with her new partner and looking very much put out that he was getting so much attention. Susannah saw her look from Neville to her new partner, and she looked a little disappointed in the new comparison.

Good for you, Nev, she thought. *Good for you. Maybe there is such a thing as second chances.*

Chris waited for Neville to retake his seat, and then he reached into his pocket, and pulled out a wad of notes.

'Neville will be here shortly, ladies, but first of all, I would like to make the first match of the day.' The crowd oohed collectively, and Susannah's heart melted. 'Susannah,' he started. He leaned down in front of her, so his elbows were on the booth counter in front of her. 'Susie. I have here in my hand a thousand pounds for the charity pot, for the chance to match with you.'

The crowd went mad, shouts of 'Go for it' and 'Grab it, you fool!' ringing out in the crowd. Chris grinned, and she found herself grinning back. Quietly, so the microphone wouldn't pick it up, she whispered to him.

'What are you doing?' she asked, half in shock, half delighted.

He leaned in close, and she caught the familiar scent of him. God, she loved this man. He was insufferable, and stubborn. Sometimes she wanted to slap him; other times she wanted to grab him and never let go. He whispered back, and she was lost for ever.

'I'm proving that, to me, you will never be second best. To anyone. Ever. You healed me, Susie. I couldn't imagine wanting to devote the rest of my life to anyone or anything else, but you. You are it for me. When you walked away, when I came to the hospice… It was all just so obvious to me once I saw it. You irritate the hell out of me, and I want you to do it for ever.' He leaned closer, and the crowd grew louder. 'I know you think I'm stubborn, and surly.'

'Don't forget oafish,' she quipped, and her lips twitched. He broke out into a broad grin.

'That too,' he acquiesced. 'I was all those things, but it wasn't just about losing Karen. It was the fact that we'd realised, too late, that our jobs were our main loves. We cared for each other, but it wasn't like this.' He pointed his finger from his chest to hers, mirroring the action she'd used on him all that time ago. 'I was meant to come here, for you. For this.' He turned and waved his arm across the crowds, who were all waiting with bated breath for her answer.

'So,' he said, putting the money in the glass

jar Cheryl had brought up, 'this money is in the pot, whatever you decide. I just want you to know that, to me, you will always come first. I love you, Susie. With my whole heart.' A single tear ran down her cheek, and he brushed it away with his hand. 'So,' he said into the microphone now, addressing the crowd once more, 'the money is in the pot, whatever you decide. Susannah Harkin, will you make me the happiest vet in the village…' he waggled his brows at her, turning her tears into laughter '…and be my match?'

The crowd went nuts, but Susannah didn't hear them. All she could see was Chris, and the whole village watching him woo her. Right there, where her parents and Heather had lived and died, where she'd grown from a girl into a woman. From a broken divorcee, to an independent woman, who now had a man who cherished the things in this simple life just as much as she did. They'd both had their hearts broken, and seen grief close enough for it to leave a mark on their souls for ever. They'd still found each other though, and she thanked her lucky stars for it. She stood up, taking the microphone from him.

'Dr Jennings,' she said, liking the feel of

his name on her lips. She wanted to shout it from the rooftops. 'I thought you'd never ask.'

The crowd went crazy, and as he pulled her close, taking her mouth with his, she could hear everyone cheer. Hendrix was going mental, zooming around the booth like an excited child and leading the dog chorus, and she could hear the yells and whoops from Cheryl, Helen and Roz even above the din of everyone else. Chris pulled her into his arms, and kissed her as if he was afraid to stop. Which was ridiculous, because one thing she would never want him to do was stop kissing her.

When they eventually pulled away, the crowd rejoiced, and Roz took the microphone, calling Neville up for his chance. As Chris came and pulled Susannah towards the house, they could just make out Nancy elbowing her way to the front of the queue, pushing the other women out of the way to be the first to get to Neville. Chris saw it too, and laughed. 'Good for you, Nev,' he said.

Once they were in the house, he pulled her in for another long kiss.

'You're mad—you know that, don't you?' she said breathlessly when he finally let them both come up for air. 'You paid a thousand quid for something you could have had for free.'

He laughed heartily. 'Ah well, it's only money. I was thinking of the tax write-off anyway.' She went to slap him on the arm, and he grabbed it, linking her fingers through his, looking down at her. She felt so seen under his gaze. So cherished. 'I would have given the shirt off my back for the chance to prove to you how much you mean to me.' Another kiss, this time on her jawline. She shuddered with delight. 'God, I wish we didn't have a million people to look after. We could have a lot of fun, just the two of us.' He lowered his lips to her neck, tracing a line of kisses along her skin to her collarbone. 'I love you so much.'

She drew back to look into his eyes. 'I love you too, Dr Moody Pants.' The look of relief and delight on his face made her love him all the more in that instant. 'I'm so glad you came to Puddle Lake.'

'Not half as glad as I am,' he replied, touching his forehead to hers as he pressed his body against hers. 'Now, what do you say, shall we get this over with? We have some dogs to save and some money to raise.' He dipped his gaze to her body. 'And tonight, I would like to revisit the wonky-top situation, if you're up for it.'

She blushed as desire and love flowed through her.

'In the interests of medical science, I'm sure that can be arranged.'

His smile lit up the room, brighter than anything she'd ever worn.

'That's what I like to hear. Let's go.' Reluctantly letting her loose from his embrace, he took her hand in his, and together they headed back out, to enjoy their special day with the villagers.

Hendrix was waiting by the door, wagging his tail in delight as he spotted the pair.

'Do you think he'll get on with Tank?' she asked. 'I adopted him.'

Chris's eyes snapped to hers, and he grinned. 'You did?'

'Yeah. I couldn't let him go, not after you saved him.'

Hendrix jumped up at them both, but Chris clicked his fingers and he settled back down.

'You know what?' He smiled. 'I have a feeling the four of us are going to get on like a house on fire.' As they headed out onto the lawn, the villagers cheered their arrival.

Chris didn't leave her side all day, and

every day after that. Susannah never felt second best again, and she would be grateful for ever for the paws and waggy tails that had brought the two of them together and helped them to find each other. They had found their for ever home, just like the furry souls they'd helped along the way.

* * * * *

*If you enjoyed this story, check out
these other great reads from
Rachel Dove*

The Paramedic's Secret Son
Fighting for the Trauma Doc's Heart

All available now!